SEXUAL DYSFUNCTION

Edited by **Berend Olivier**

Sexual Dysfunction
http://dx.doi.org/10.5772/63284
Edited by Berend Olivier

Contributors

Pedro J Tarraga Lopez, Angel Celada, Jose Antonio Rodriguez Montes, Carmen Celada, Berend Olivier, Jocelien D.A. Olivier, Diana C. Esquivel Franco, Marcel Waldinger, Dana I Stoian, Marius Craina, Adalbert Schiller, Puiu Velea, Corina Paul, Mihaela Craciunescu, Ioana Mozos, Götz Egloff

Published by InTech

Janeza Trdine 9, 51000 Rijeka, Croatia

Publishing Process Manager Dajana Pemac
Technical Editor SPi Global
Cover InTech Design team

First published June, 2017
Printed in Croatia
Legal deposit, Croatia: National and University Library in Zagreb

Additional hard copies can be obtained from orders@intechopen.com

Sexual Dysfunction, Edited by Berend Olivier
p. cm.
Print ISBN 978-953-51-3263-9
Online ISBN 978-953-51-3264-6

For EU product safety concerns:
IN TECH d.o.o., Prolaz Marije Krucifikse Kozulić 3, 51000 Rijeka, Croatia,
info@intechopen.com or visit our website at intechopen.com.

Meet the editor

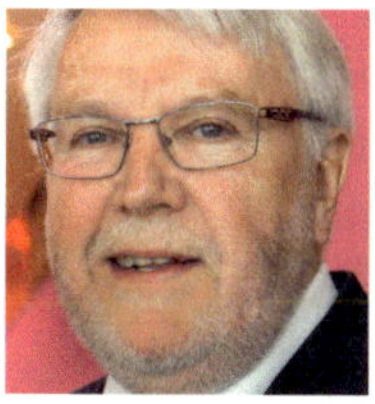

Berend Olivier studied biology and got his PhD degree in Neurobiology at Groningen University. He worked for 22 years at Solvay Pharmaceuticals leading active research and development of psychoactive drugs, including antidepressants, antipsychotics and anxiolytics and a new group of drugs, serenics, aiming for reduction of pathological aggression. He was involved in research and development around fluvoxamine, a marketed SSRI antidepressant, anxiolytic and anti-OCD medicine. In 1999, he worked for 2 years in New York to set up a biotech start-up, PsychoGenics Inc., developing animal psychiatric and neurological (genetic) models in order to screen and find new psychoactive molecules. From 1992–2014, he was a professor of CNS Pharmacology at Utrecht University, performing research on animal models, brain mechanisms and pharmacology of psychiatric disorders.

Contents

Preface

The Diagnostic and Statistical Manual of Mental Disorders (DSM-5) describes a plethora of sexual dysfunctions in males and females illustrating the diversity and heterogeneity of sexual disorders. The characterization of a sexual dysfunction is a complex issue needing extensive clinical, psychological and psychiatric expertise to come to a reliable diagnosis and includes many factors including partner, individual vulnerability and genetic, cultural, religious and several medical factors. Sexual functioning and dysfunctioning involve complex interactions of biological, sociocultural and psychological factors. In any case, problems caused by interfering factors, like drugs, medicines, medical conditions or external stressors, should be excluded before making a dedicated diagnosis.

The present volume illustrates various aspects involved in sexual (dys)functioning showing the breadth of the field. Chapter 1 gives an introductory view on the field, introduces the various chapters and shortly discusses progress in premature ejaculation and female sexual interest and arousal disorder. Chapter 2 deals with an important male sexual problem, erectile dysfunction. Apart from an overview of the problems and causes of erectile dysfunctions, an extensive study is described where patients with various cardiovascular risks were assessed on erectile problems using an extensive range of variables analyzed. Not surprisingly, a high incidence of erectile dysfunction was found in patients with high cardiovascular risk factors. Interestingly, erectile dysfunction improved more if these cardiovascular risk factors were strictly controlled. Such a study illustrates the importance of lifestyle factors in the sexual well-being of males. In Chapter 3, an impressive overview is given on the role of testosterone and particularly the lack or diminished levels of testosterone (hypogonadism) in every aspect of sexual development and life. Ageing appears an important factor that is associated with a gradual decrease in the amount of testosterone produced, and also lifestyle (obesity, metabolic syndrome, and the use of anabolic steroids) may lead to hypogonadism and associated sexual dysfunctions and complaints. In Chapter 4, sexual dysfunctions occurring during major depression are discussed. Several sexual problems occur both in male- and female-depressed patients. Many antidepressants and particularly selective serotonin reuptake inhibitors (SSRIs) induce sexual side effects in depressed patients that further deteriorate the often-already present sexual problems. This is one of the main reasons of treatment cessation. New antidepressants lacking these sexual side effects are badly needed. The contribution describes an animal model in rodents with predictive and face validity towards human (male) sexual behaviour and sensitivity towards sexual side effects of potential antidepressants. Development of new antidepressants without such (sexual) side effects is a time-consuming and costly trajectory, but it is expected that such medication will become available in the next decade. In the final chapter, a nice overview is given of circumcision and the ideas, rituals and beliefs about its function. There are many opinions about the role of circumcision in sexual functioning and dysfunctioning, and the chapter nicely explains a lot of ideas and opinions on these items, including psychological, religious and medical theories. It gives a welcome, broad overview of the many aspects involved in thinking about sex and its dysfunctions.

Professor Dr. Berend Olivier
Professor Emeritus
Pharmacology of the Central Nervous System
Faculty of Sciences, Department of Psychopharmacology
Utrecht University, Utrecht, the Netherlands

Adjunct Professor
Department of Psychiatry
Yale University School of Medicine
New Haven, USA

Section 1

Sexual Dysfunction: Introduction and Perspective

Chapter 1

Introductory Chapter: Sexual Dysfunction - Introduction and Perspective

Berend Olivier

Additional information is available at the end of the chapter

http://dx.doi.org/10.5772/intechopen.69092

The fifth *Diagnostic and Statistical Manual of Mental Disorders* (DSM-5) of the American Psychiatric Association [1] gives the following classifications of sexual dysfunctions: delayed ejaculation, erectile disorder, female orgasmic disorder, female sexual interest/arousal disorder, genito-pelvic pain/penetration disorder, male hypoactive sexual desire disorder, premature (early) ejaculation, substance-/medication-induced sexual dysfunction, other specified sexual dysfunction, and unspecified sexual dysfunction. It is evident that sexual dysfunctions constitute a heterogeneous group of disorders. They are characterized by clinically significant disturbances to respond sexually or experience sexual pleasure. Determining the character of the sexual dysfunction is a complex issue, which needs extensive clinical and psychological/psychiatric expertise in order to come to a correct clinical judgment and includes partner and relationship factors, individual vulnerability, psychiatric comorbidity, stressors, and cultural, religious, and medical factors.

Sexual functioning involves a complex interaction of biological, sociocultural, and psychological factors, which makes a clear diagnosis sometimes rather difficult. In any case, problems should be ruled out that are caused by interfering factors, like drugs, medicines, a medical condition (e.g., pelvic nerve damage) or external factors like partner violence, or other severe stressors.

In the present volume, four chapters are included that represent various aspects involved in sexual behavior and its dysfunctions in a very broad sense. These chapters also give a window on the complex issues involved in normal and dysfunctional sexual interactions.

In Chapter 2, the focus is on erectile disorder or erectile dysfunction. Erectile dysfunction (ED) is defined as a disorder that is characterized by the incapacity to sufficiently achieve and maintain an erection in order to enjoy a satisfactory sexual relationship. After premature ejaculation, it is the most frequent sexual dysfunction in men. Erectile disorder is frequently, but not always, associated with cardiovascular risk factors, and the authors describe and discuss an elegant study in Spain, using a very extensive tool of methods and measures on a large cohort of males. The results indicate a high prevalence of erectile dysfunction in patients with high vascular risks. Improvement in erectile dysfunction was clearly associated with improved control of these cardiovascular risk factors. The study nicely illustrates the complexities involved in erectile problems and also in the difficulties in treating them properly. Moreover, the authors discuss the various factors that influence erectile functions like aging, lifestyle (smoking, diet), high blood pressure, atherosclerosis, and blood pressure medications. Although modifying lifestyle risk factors may help, in many cases patients also need medications to improve or correct erectile problems [2]. Phosphodiesterase type 5 inhibitors (PDE5i) have revolutionized ED treatment, although there are limitations in their use (e.g., diabetes and nerve injury patients often respond poorly to PDE5i). In the last decade, several new treatment strategies for the treatment of ED have been pursued, aiming at treating underlying microvascular abnormalities, restoring smooth muscle contractility, preventing cavernosal fibrosis, promoting endothelial revascularization, modulating neurohumoral pathways, and regenerating new penile tissue [3].

Hypogonadism is the decrease or absence of hormonal secretion from the gonads. In males, this condition is called androgen deficiency and is characterized by a decrease or absence of testosterone (T) secretion from the testes. T plays an essential role in normal male development starting from the very early stage in life (intrauterine) and is necessary for the emergence and maintenance of many male characteristics and functions, including body mass, bone density, libido, potency, and spermatogenesis. It is also indispensable for normal sexual functioning in adult life, and in puberty T is extremely important for a mature male phenotype at somatic and genital areas in the body. In Chapter 3, by Stolan and coworkers, an extensive overview is given on the role of T levels in normal sexual life and the dramatic effects of the consequences of hypogonadism, i.e., low T levels. Not only classical hypogonadic types, due to testicular disease or caused by central nervous system-, hypothalamic-, or hypophyseal-induced hypogonadism are described, but also the important partial T deficiency coinciding with aging is discussed. Apart from those, not only secondary T deficiency may occur due to problems associated with enhanced body weight (frequently seen in diabetes and metabolic syndrome) but also hypogonadism due to the chronic use of anabolic steroids or after long and intense stress exposure, even in young men. The authors describe therapeutic approaches to each kind of hypogonadism, based on individualized treatment including lifestyle changes, weight loss, exercising, and supplemental therapy. Because normal testosterone levels play a decisive role in various aspects of daily sex life, like daily sexual day dreaming or sexual fantasies, it is extremely evident how important normal T levels are for male sexual well-being. It can be easily seen that hypogonadism may lead to various complaints in daily life and in particular sexual complaints.

Mood disorders, and in particular major depression, are very often associated with sexual dysfunctions, both in male and in female patients. Such sexual dysfunctions cover the whole domain of sexual problems including libido, delayed ejaculations, erectile, and orgasmic disturbances. When major depression needs urgent treatment with an antidepressant, the latter often (and particularly with serotonergic antidepressants like selective serotonin reuptake inhibitors (SSRIs) and selective serotonin-norepinephrine reuptake inhibitors (SNRIs)) comes with additional sexual side effects. This makes the situation for the patient often unbearable and frequently leads to ceasing the treatment. In Chapter 4 (Olivier and coworkers), the various factors that are involved in the complex interaction between the primary disorder (major depression) and the unwanted sexual dysfunctions (both caused by the disease itself and by the sexual side effects of the antidepressant) are described, primarily focused on men (mainly because the female domain is less well investigated). It appears extremely difficult to disentangle the intrinsic sexual problems associated with depression from those induced by the antidepressant. Sexual dysfunctions remain one of the important reasons to noncompliance to the drug treatment, even if the depressive mood is lifted and the patient feels better. One of the big challenges for research of new antidepressants is the design and development of such compounds without sexual side effects, although other side effects should also be avoided if possible. There is an ongoing heavy discussion on the therapeutic efficacy of antidepressants (and all other psychotropic agents) and their side effects [4]. This discussion and its implications make it very clear that we lack fundamental insight in the cause of psychiatric diseases (including depression) and that fundamental research into the mechanisms of action of "normal" functioning should lead to insight into pathological functioning. Only then, it might be possible to design and develop new psychotropic drugs, including antidepressants that are true "medicines" instead of drugs that merely treat "symptoms." Fundamental research of the brain is often difficult to perform directly in man, and animal research can be of utmost importance, although always caution should be used in the translation from animal to man because of sometimes large species differences. Chapter 4 also describes such an approach for sexual side effects of (novel) antidepressants. Because sexual side effects of antidepressants, at least in men, are relatively well described in the literature [5], those antidepressants can be used in a translational animal model that is sensitive to sexual side effects. The rat model reflects several aspects of the sexual side effects of classical antidepressants (tricyclics, SSRIs, SNRIs, NRIs), including delayed onset of action and disappearing of the sexual side effects after stopping treatment. Two recently introduced antidepressants vilazodone and vortioxetine, according to clinical studies [6, 7], exert no or less sexual side effects in depressed patients compared to classic antidepressants, especially the SSRIs. These two compounds had no sexual side effects in the rat model of sexual behavior used in Chapter 4. The model has considerable translational validity and can and will be used for future studies into sexual side effects of new antidepressants. Moreover, the model can also be used for fundamental research into the brain mechanisms and circuitry underlying sexual behavior. Understanding the normal functioning and inducing perturbations in this circuitry might help in finding new ways to treat side effects of novel and "real" psychotropic medicines.

A topic not dealt with in the present contributions but related to the use of antidepressants and the sexual inhibitory effects of the latter (notably the SSRIs) is premature ejaculation, one of the sexual dysfunctions mentioned in DSM-5. Premature ejaculation (PE) has been defined as persistent or recurrent ejaculation occurring during partnered sexual activity within approx. 1 minute following vaginal penetration and before the person wishes it. PE must be present for at least 6 months and must be present on practically all occasions of sexual activity and causes clinically significant distress in the individual. PE cannot be better explained by a nonsexual mental disorder or as a consequence of a severe relationship distress or other major stressors and is not caused by the effects of a substance/medication or another medical condition. PE can be lifelong or acquired, generalized, or situational and may have mild (intravaginal ejaculation latency time (IELT) of 30–60 seconds), moderate (IELT of 15–30 seconds), or severe (IELT<15 seconds) effects. Treatment by selective serotonin reuptake inhibitors (SSRIs) has really led to a paradigm shift in the understanding and treatment of PE as all SSRIs exert ejaculation delaying effects in men with PE [8, 9]. Although the treatment of PE by SSRIs is "off-label," it is the present therapy used for PE, notwithstanding the nonsexual side effects and the need to take the medication daily and permanently [10]. An ideal anti-PE medication would be "on demand," that can be taken shortly (hours) before sexual activity. Although it still would come with side effects, it is assumed that many men may prefer the convenience of "on demand" dosing compared to daily and long-term dosing [11]. The search for an "on demand" treatment for PE has led to the development of dapoxetine, which has received approval for treatment of PE in many countries, although it has not been approved by the US Food and Drug Administration (FDA). Dapoxetine is a potent SSRI, and it is postulated that its rapid absorption and rapid appearance of peak plasma concentration combined with a relatively short half-life lead to an ideal pharmacokinetic profile for such an "on demand" profile. Dapoxetine has some minor "on demand" efficacy but clearly is not a breakthrough medicine in the treatment of PE [11]. Another SSRI, with a comparable profile as dapoxetine, DA-8031 is in development for PE, but efficacy data have not yet been elucidated [12, 13]. Several other approaches for treatment of PE are used or are in development, including local anesthetics (e.g., lidocaine) used as cream, gel, or spray, and are moderately effective in delaying ejaculation [10]. Several other compounds with various mechanisms of action (tramadol, α_1-adrenoceptor antagonists, oxytocin antagonists, modafinil, and botulin-A toxin) have been proposed in the treatment of PE but need extensive testing and will not reach the market soon.

Treatment of female sexual dysfunction lags behind the available male treatments (ED, PE, hypogonadism). Low sexual desire is the most common sexual complaint in women, and many females suffer from sexual dissatisfaction that often negatively interferes with quality of life. Initially, these sexual complaints were classified as hypoactive sexual desire disorder (HSDD) but have merged in DSM-5 with female sexual arousal disorder (FSAD) into the diagnosis of female sexual interest/arousal disorder (FSIAD). Most research up to now has been using HSDD as the most common sexual dysfunction disorder that affects many women all over the world. A recent study in the USA found that more than 7% of US women suffer from HSDD [14]. In 2012, the FDA approved flibanserin (Addyi™) for the treatment of premenstrual women with HSDD. Flibanserin is a 5-HT_{1A} receptor agonist and 5-HT_{2A} receptor antagonist and has moderate pro-sexual activities [15]. Several other hormonal (testosterone) and pharmacological (buspirone, bupropion) drugs have been tested but have not led yet to approved pharmacotherapy for FSIAD. Currently, two drugs are under investigation for the treatment of FSIAD that combine a low dose of sublingual testosterone with either a PDE5i (sildenafil) or a partial 5-HT_{1A} receptor agonist (buspirone) [16]. Sublingual T is rapidly absorbed, induces a rapid peak in T, and is eliminated within 2–3 h [16]. However, T induces an increase in sexual motivation 3–6 h after administration (therapeutic window). Administration of either sildenafil or buspirone in such a way that their therapeutic window coincides with that induced by T leads to rather strong pro-sexual effects [16]. The (T + PDE5i) treatment (Lybrido) appears particularly active in women with HSDD/FSIAD due to a relatively insensitive system for sexual cues and the (T + buspirone) treatment (Lybridos) for

HSDD/FSIAD women due to dysfunctional activation of sexual inhibitory mechanisms [16]. In a small study in women with SSRI-induced sexual dysfunction, both drug combinations also showed promising results [17]. Further development of these promising drugs will take time, but at least it indicates the possibility to develop efficient and innovative pharmacotherapy for for FSIAD. Another potential medicine for FSIAD might come from influencing a completely different mechanism of action by bremelanotide, an agonist of melanocortin 3 (MC_3) and MC_4 receptors. Preliminary data are promising, but again further development need to show clear pro-sexual activity [15]. The positive message from all these developments is that the lack of effective medications to treat female sexual dysfunctions seems to come to an end.

Finally, in the last chapter by Egloff, various aspects of circumcision are described and discussed in a broad context. Biomedical, psychosomatic, psychotherapeutic, cultural, religious, clinical, and pharmacological aspects of circumcision are portrayed. The function of the foreskin, e.g., hygiene or protection of the glans penis, in normal (sexual) life is discussed, as well as in a clinical setting. Whether circumcision influences sexual behavior or may lead to sexual dysfunction, or, in contrast, improves sexual dysfunctions, is a matter of debate but certainly needs more research. The beauty of this chapter is that it adds a lot of additional facts and thoughts about the complexity of human sexuality.

Author details

Berend Olivier

Address all correspondence to: b.olivier@uu.nl

1 Groningen Institute for Evolutionary Life Sciences (GELIFES), Faculty of Science and Engineering, Rijksuniversiteit Groningen, Groningen, The Netherlands

2 Department of Psychopharmacology, Science Faculty, Utrecht University, The Netherlands

3 Department of Psychiatry, Yale University School of Medicine, New Haven, USA

References

[1] American Psychiatric Association. Diagnostic and Statistical Manual of Mental Disorders, 5th ed. Arlington, VA: American Psychiatric Association, 2013

[2] Clina S, Cohen DJ, Vieira M. Diagnosis of erectile dysfunction. Current Opinion in Psychiatry. 2014;**27**:394-399

[3] Decaluwé K, Pauwels B, Boydens C, van de Voorde J. Treatment of erectile dysfunction: New targets and strategies from recent research. Pharmacology Biochemistry and Behavior. 2014;**121**:146-157

[4] Gøtzsche. Deadly Psychiatry and Organized Denial. København: People's Press; 2015

[5] Segraves RT, Balon R. Antidepressant-induced sexual dysfunction in men. Pharmacology Biochemistry and Behavior. 2014;**121**:132-137

[6] Sahli ZT, Banerjee P, Tarazi FI. The preclinical and clinical effects of Vilazodone for the treatment of major depressive disorder. Expert Opinion on Drug Discovery. 2016;**11**: 515-523

[7] Connolly KR, Thase ME. Vortioxetine: A new treatment for major depressive disorder. Expert Opinion on Pharmacotherapy. 2016;**17**:421-431

[8] Waldinger MD, Zwinderman AH, Schweitzer DH, Olivier B. Relevance of methodological design for the interpretation of efficacy of drug treatment of premature ejaculation: A systematic review and meta-analysis. International Journal of Impotence Research. 2004;**16**:369-381

[9] Gur S, Kadowitz PJ, Sikka SC. Current therapies for premature ejaculation. Drug Discovery Today. 2016;**21**:1147-1154

[10] McMahon CG. Emerging and investigational drugs for premature ejaculation. Translational Andrology and Urology. 2016;**5**:487-501

[11] Waldinger MD, Schweitzer DH. Premature ejaculation and pharmaceutical company-based medicine: The dapoxetine case. The Journal of Sexual Medicine. 2008;**5**:966-997

[12] Jeon HJ, Kim HS, Lee CH, Lee YG, Choi SM, Sohn YS, Shin CY, Kim J, Shim HJ, Kang KK, Ahn BO, Kim SH. Candidate molecule for premature ejaculation, DA-8031: In vivo and in vitro characterization of DA-8031. Urology. 2011;**77**:1006.e17-1006.e21

[13] Shin D, Lee S, Yi S, Yoon SH, Cho JY, Bahng MY, Jang IJ, Yu KS. Pharmacokinetics and tolerability of DA-8031, a novel selective serotonin reuptake inhibitor for premature ejaculation in healthy male subjects. Drug Design, Development and Therapy. 2017;**11**:713-723

[14] Rosen RC, Connor MK, Miyasato G, Link C, Shifren JL, Fisher WA, Derogatis LR, Schobelock MJ. Sexual desire problems in women seeking healthcare: A novel study design for ascertaining prevalence of hypoactive sexual desire disorder in clinic-based samples of U.S. women. Journal of Women's Health. 2012;**21**:505-515

[15] Kingsberg SA, Clayton AH, Pfaus JG. The female sexual response: Current models, neurobiological underpinnings and agents currently approved or under investigation for the treatment of hypoactive sexual desire disorder. CNS Drugs. 2015;**29**:915-933

[16] Poels S, Bloemers J, van Rooij K, Koppeschaar H, Olivier B, Tuiten A. Two novel combined drug treatments for women with hypoactive sexual desire disorder. Pharmacology Biochemistry and Behavior. 2014;**121**:71-79

[17] van Rooij K, Poels S, Worst P, Bloemers J, Koppeschaar H, Goldstein A, Olivier B, Tuiten A. Efficacy of testosterone combined with a PDE5 inhibitor and testosterone combined with a serotonin (1A) receptor agonist in women with SSRI-induced sexual dysfunction. A preliminary study. European Journal of Pharmacology. 2015;**753**:246-251

Section 2

Erectile Dysfunction

Chapter 2

Erectile Dysfunction Associated with Cardiovascular Risk Factors

Ángel Celada Rodríguez, Pedro Juan Tárraga López,
José Antonio Rodríguez Montes,
Ma Loreto Tarraga Marcos and
Carmen Celada Roldan

Additional information is available at the end of the chapter

http://dx.doi.org/10.5772/intechopen.69104

Abstract

Objectives: (1) Determine erectile dysfunction (ED) prevalence in patients with cardiovascular risk factors (CVRF). (2) Assess ED incidence in relation to the extent of controlling CVRF. Methodology: Patients: Enrolled participants came to the health centres in the study area. In accordance with the incidence of diseases with cardiovascular risks (CVR) in the Basic Health Regions of the study area, sample size was calculated with a 95% confidence interval and an alpha error of 0.005, resulting in a sample of 210 people, of which 30 could not complete the study for various reasons (change of address, death, refused to complete questionnaire, etc.). A full awareness and diffusion campaign was organized with talks and leaflets. Letters: A standard letter was given to patients which explained the importance of sexual health, offering them an appointment with a DUE (Diploma in Nursing) survey taker. The questionnaire was devised by the research group and was given by a fully trained DUE survey taker. Previously, contact was made with all the health centres, physicians and nursing staff to give them information on ED and CVRF and to inform them about the work to be done in their health region. Those patients who did not come to the appointment were telephoned to insist on the importance of attending and completing the questionnaire. Variables analysis: We analysed age, level of education, civil status, height, weight and body mass index (BMI), SBP, DBP, smoking habit, number cigarettes/day, year smoking began, ex-smoker, year smoking stopped, alcohol consumption, grams alcohol/week, as well as consumption of other drugs, frequency and type. Blood test: glucose, haemoglobin glycated haemoglobin, total cholesterol, LDL cholesterol, HDL cholesterol, triglycerides, artherogenic index, creatinine, urea, GOT, GPT, gamma-GT and PSA. Urine test: micro-albuminuria, proteinuria and creatinine clearance. ECG. Diabetes diagnosed at least 1 year ago and prescribed drugs to treat it. High blood pressure diagnosed at least 1 year ago and prescribed drugs to treat it. Dyslipidaemia (hypercholesterolaemia) diagnosed at least 1 year ago and prescribed drugs to treat it. Concomitant diseases of at least 1 year and drugs (up to 3)

SHIM questionnaire and ED according to SHIM. Statistical analysis: an observational, descriptive, analytical, cross-sectional study. Qualitative variables are presented as exact values and a percentage; quantitative variables as the mean and standard deviation (SD). A means comparison was done with the Student's *t*-test for independent groups, or the Mann-Whitney U test if normality conditions (using the Kolmogorov-Smirnoff or Shapiro-Wilks test) were not fulfilled. The chi-squared test was used for qualitative variables. Results: Of the 210 selected people, 179 completed the questionnaire (85.2%). The mean age was 64.5 ± 11.6 years. When analysing all the study variables in relation to the main variable, presence or absence of ED, age played an important role in ED appearing as ED incidence rises with age. Blood pressure had no significant relationship with the studied variable, and the same hold for BMI and its subdivision into normal weight and obesity. As regards toxic habits, neither cigarette smoking nor alcohol consumption influenced the presence of ED. The same hold for the sociological-type variables (civil states, level of education). Regarding the biochemical variables from blood tests, a significant relationship with the atherogenic index and its recoded variable at high and low atherogenic risk ($p < 0.04$) was noted. In the glycaemic profile, a glycaemia mean of 126 mg/dl was obtained in the ED presence group, which is the cut-off point proposed by ADA117 (American Diabetes Association) to consider a subject diabetic. Likewise, glycated haemoglobin presented figures in the two groups can be considered an alternation of a practically diabetic glucose metabolism. In our study, the presence of diabetic disease, high blood pressure (HBP) and dyslipidaemia showed no significant relationship with ED presence for each disease. However, in the combination of these diseases, a statistically significant relationship was seen when CVR increases, according to the Framinghan tables. Neither did each disease's duration show a significant relationship with ED presence nor significant differences for the drugs used to treat the three pathologies were found. The coronary risk calculated according to the Framinghan tables indicated a statistically significant result, as did excessive risk (the difference between the coronary risk and the average assigned per age) for ED presence. The LISAT 8 test suggested that ED affected health-associated quality of life and was statistically significant in two items of sex life and economic situation and was borderline statistically significant in the general life and working life items. Conclusions: There is a high ED prevalence in patients with high CVR. When ED improves, the better CVRFs are controlled. These patients' pluripathology implies aggressive polymedication which doctors must consider as it increases the risk of ED.

Keywords: erectile dysfunction, cardiovascular risk, primary health care

1. Introduction

Erectile dysfunction (ED) is defined as a disorder characterized by the incapacity to sufficiently achieve and maintain an erection to enjoy a sexual relation and is, after premature ejaculation, the most common form of sexual dysfunction among men. The term 'erectile dysfunction' is recommended instead of 'impotence' because it defines the problem more accurately and has less social connotations [1–3].

Most cases are of an organic origin frequently owing to vascular diseases that diminish the blood flow to the penis, but can also be the result of psychological, neurological, hormonal, cavernous alterations, combinations of these and even cultural-type factors [2–4].

The first known reliable population data available are those of Kinsey's report dating back to 1948, in which 15,781 males aged 10–80 years participated who were stratified by ages, education and residence, of which only 4108 adults were assessed (older than 25 years), with half of these aged over 35 years and only 356 aged above 55 years. Therefore, conclusions are representative of males up to the age of 55 years and must be interpreted with caution for older populations. According to Kinsey's report, ED affects less than 1% of the population aged under 30 years; less than 35% of the population up to the age of 45 years; and 6.7% of those aged 45–55 years; 25% of those over the age of 65 years, and up to 75% in males above the age of 80 years [3–6].

In 1994, the Massachusetts Male Aging Study (MMAS) was published, which studied a population of 1270 American males aged 40–70 years. Among its results, it is worth stressing an ED prevalence of 52 ± 1.23% (9.6% complete, 25.2% moderate, 17.2% minimum) and a 5% risk of suffering ED at the age of 40 years, which triples to 15% at the age of 70 years [6].

In 1996, the first epidemiological study in Spain, known by the Spanish acronym EDEM (Study into Male ED), was conducted with an ED-based population. It included 2476 males aged between 25 and 70 years, and a simple overall self-assessment question to categorize subjects with ED, as well as the IEFI's (International Index of Erectile Function) erectile function domain. ED prevalence rate in our country is 12.1% according to the simple question and 19% according to the IEFI's erectile function domain. After making population-based estimations according to the corrected 1991 census, the number of Spanish males with some degree of ED ranges between 1 and 1.5 million, of whom around 850,000 have moderate or serious/complete ED [6].

In 2002, a study appeared which was performed as part of Primary Health Care in Spain (Guirao Sánchez, the APLAUDE study) [7], with a sample of 125 patients. It discovered that two out of every three patients with ED had associated illnesses, and that one out of three was not aware of his health problem. The control of chronic diseases improved significantly, and three out of every four patients responded to sildenafil.

Presence of sexual alterations is frequent in cases of high blood pressure [8–14], and hypertensive patients can be considered individuals with a higher likelihood of becoming impotent as they face a triple threat: hypertension itself can diminish the production of neurotransmitters involved in erection; arterial consequences of hypertension that alter the arterial wall and hypertension treatment may alter the erectile cycle.

The effect that hypertension has on the arterial wall is known and exercised at two levels: diminishing arterial elasticity and being capable of causing endothelial lesion. In all bifurcations of the arterial system, hypertension causes 'uprooting' of endothelial cells owing to increased blood flow clashing against the vascular wall. After every endothelial repair, these predilation zones become increasingly prone to new endothelial lesions since the structures exposed in each endothelial lesion induce platelets to cover the lesion [12–14].

Many medicines are able to altering men's sexual function at different levels. Anti-hypertensives are the main cause of medicine-related impotence. They may cause impotence because they lower perfusion pressure at the cavernous hypogastric arterial level. The most common drugs are methyldopa or clonidine, which act at two levels: centrally, by diminishing sexual desire, and peripherally, by making erection difficult. Apart from these sympatholythics (including guanethidine, reserpine), alpha blockers, MAOI (nialamide) and vasodilators (hydralazine), beta blockers and diuretics, which are often used in combination in almost 15–30% of treated individuals, also may cause impotence.

It is necessary to bear in mind that anti-hypertensives are, in many cases, only a triggering factor and reveals a latent lesion. This occurs when atheromatous lesions exist in penis arteries, which on itself are not sufficient to alter erection but may cause impotence when combined with a treatment that drops blood pressure and withdraws blood [12–17].

Sexual impotence affects diabetics [12–16] at an estimated percentage of between 30 and 50%. It is important to stress that impotence is established in most cases in the year before the disease evolves. Nonetheless, and whatever the cause, diabetes causes 50% of cases of erectile alterations after it has gradually evolved over a 10-year period. The cause is multifactorial, but arterial and neuronal lesions clearly predominate. An arterial lesion is not necessarily found in the presence of neuronal lesions.

In one study, the prevalence of risk factors in 440 individuals with ED [14], 30% diabetics were found. This implies that diabetes is significantly more common in the ED population than in the general population for similarly aged individuals.

Diabetic microangiopathy significantly diminishes arteries' diameter (calibre) and reduces the blood flow required for erection. This is due to lesions forming that affect not only micro-vessels, but also surrounding interstitial tissue.

Disturbances in the bloodstream induced by diabetes also intervene in circulation alterations at the micro-circulation level, along with structural alterations of this micro-circulation. This phenomenon is linked to a higher proteins rate in the acute phase where fibrinogen is the most important of these proteins.

The vegetative neuropathy of diabetes affects the parasympathic medullary centres conditioning vesical atony and ED, since these are centres common to urination and erection [14].

Former studies have demonstrated that atherogenesis is responsible for LDL cholesterol although, in parallel, HDL cholesterol acts as a protector. Total cholesterol, therefore, reflects cholesterol in various lipoproteins, of which two factors play an opposing role in vascular diseases genesis [16–18].

Lipids' isolated or associated role in altering the metabolism in terms of participating in the organic disorder of ED is an important one, be it less significant than the action of tobacco or diabetes. Total cholesterol appears to play a more important role than triglycerides in the pathogenicity of lipid-caused metabolism alterations in ED. Its rate increases with age in individuals whose alteration has an arterial component.

Despite its high prevalence and unquestionable impact on men's self-esteem and quality of life, ED is still under-diagnosed owing to the social and cultural environment that leads to fear and shame to consult it. In the next part, we describe a study into many factors probably involved in the prevalence of ED.

1.1. An observational, descriptive, analytical, cross-sectional study

The study was initiated at primary care in the area of Albacete county (Spain), in rural area as well as in an urban area. Three health centres participated in total.

The enrolled participants included in this study were those who visited the health centres.

In accordance with the cardiovascular risk (CVR) diseases incidence in the basic health regions of the study area [36], sample size was calculated with a 95% confidence interval and an alpha error of 0.005, which resulted in a sample of 210 people, of which 30 finally did not complete the study for various reasons (change of address, death, refusal to complete the questionnaire, etc.). The sample was chosen from the population in the basic health regions of the study area with CVR diseases.

Adequate awareness and diffusion tasks were carried out in the study population by means of:

1. Awareness talks: Three awareness talks were organised on ED to the population of Albacete.
2. Leaflets.
3. Letters: A standard type letter was given to patients which explained the importance of sexual health, and they were asked to an appointment with the DUE survey taker.

The questionnaire was devised by the research group and was conducted by a trained DUE survey taker.

A letter of presentation was sent by the research team informing about the work project to be conducted in the provinces of Albacete and Cuenca.

A second letter was sent inviting people to an appointment at their respective health centre on a given date and at a given time.

The research team and survey takers (DUE) met on several occasions to detail and plan the work. The time to perform the fieldwork took 6 months.

Previously, contact was made with all the health centres, doctors and nurses, offering them information via a colloquium on ED and CVRF and to inform them about the work to be done in their health region.

Those patients who did not come to the appointment were telephoned to insist on the importance of going to the appointment and completing the questionnaire.

Questionnaires were conducted in the time and manner agreed upon for their analysis.

The results obtained from the questionnaires were read by the research team to avoid any reading bias (see **Tables 1** and **2**).

Quantitative variables	Absence ED	Presence ED	p
Age (years), average (SD)	54.8 (10.97)	66.96 (10.38)	0.000*
BMI (kg/m^2), average (SD)	30.3 (3.5)	29.01 (3.9)	0.18
Blood pressure	137.03 (20.9)	137.3 (10.12)	0.91
PAS (mm/hg), average (DE)	80.9 (10.1)	80.2 (9.05)	0.69
PAD	56.1 (19.11)	57.2 (16.1)	0.74
TA differential			
Cigarettes/day: average (SD)	18 (11.9)	15.25 (9.9)	0.45
Packs/year: average (SD)	23.5 (16)	29.7 (19.8)	0.42
Years smoking: average (SD)	35.1 (10.3)	42.4 (12.1)	0.1
Age start smoking: average (SD)	17 (4.5)	19,5 (8.4)	0.34
Grams/week alcohol: average (SD)	154.6 (109.3)	139.1 (110.4)	0.55
Glycemia: (mg/dl), average (SD)	120.5 (40.9)	126.5 (48.3)	0.59
Glycated haemoglobin, average (SD)	6.3 (1.5)	6.6 (1.5)	0.37
Total cholesterol: (mg/dl), average (SD)	208.3 (39.4)	205.5 (39.5)	0.7
LDL-cholesterol: (mg/dl), average (SD)	130.3 (33.1)	127.9 (34.9)	0.7
HDL-cholesterol: (mg/dl), average (SD)	46.9 (10,7)	51.8 (12.5)	0.034*
No HDL cholesterol: (mg/dl), average (SD)	161.4 (40.3)	153,8 (41.1)	0.3
Triglycerides: (mg/dl), average (SD)	170.7 (70,9)	144.5 (112)	0.3
Atherogenic index: average (SD)	4.7 (1.3)	4.2 (1.3)	0.047*
Creatinine: (mg/dl), average (SD)	1.00 (0.2)	0.99 (0.2)	0.8
Uric acid: (mg/dl), average (SD)	5.9 (1.5)	5.6 (1.5)	0.37
Urea: (mg/dl), average (SD)	39.4 (14.1)	41.2 (10.0)	0.5
SGOT: (U/L), average (SD)	27.1 (9.8)	22.8 (12.3)	0.15
SGPT: (U/L): average (SD)	34.7 (19.0)	23.3 (12.1)	0.001*
Gamma-GT: (U/L), average (SD)	63.2 (110.9)	29.8 (15.5)	0.008*
PSA: (ng/ml), average (SD)	2.4 (3.7)	2.9 (4.0)	0,8
MAU:	15.4 (31.7)	6.5 (8.0)	0.1
Proteinuria:	0.07 (0.2)	3.16 (16.9)	0.6
Score LISAT-8: average (SD)	39.4 (6,1)	32.6 (7.0)	0.000*
Diabetes last: (years), average (SD)	6.8 (4.8)	9.3 (8.2)	0.11
HTA last: (years), average (SD)	6.6 (4.8)	10.5 (10.0)	0.17
Dyslipidemia last: (years), average (SD)	6.1 (6.5)	7.4 (5.5)	0.5
Coronary risk (Framinghan)	36 (20.5%)	140 (79.5%)	0.033*
Risk excess (differ between coronary risk and average risk)	36 (20.5%)	140 (79.5%)	0.012*

*$p < 0.05$: statistically significant.

Table 1. Description of variables in relation to the main variable: ED (presence or absence) in the sample surveyed.

http://dx.doi.org/10.5772/intechopen.69104

Variables	Absence ED	Presence ED	p
Age groups			
31–55 years	19 (50%)	19 (50%)	0.000*
56–70 years	14 (17.5%)	66 (82.5%)	
71–86 years	3 (4.9%)	58 (95.1%)	
Civil status			
Married	26 (19.4%)	108 (80.6%)	0.6
Living single	6 (24%)	19 (76%)	
Studies			
No studies	6 (15.4%)	33 (84.6%)	0.23
Primary studies	9 (14.1%)	55 (85.9%)	
Others	7 (29.2%)	17 (70.8%)	
BMI			
Normoweight	16 (25%)	48 (75%)	0.22
Obesity	20 (17.4%)	95 (82.6%)	
Tobacco consumption			
No	7 (17.5%)	33 (82.5%)	0.39
Daily	12 (27.3%)	32 (72.7%)	
Ex-smoker	17 (17.9%)	78 (82.1%)	
Type of ex-smoker			
1–5 years	6 (28.6%)	15 (71.4%)	0.2
Over 5 years	11 (15.5%)	60 (84.5%)	
Alcohol consumption			
Nothing	13 (18.8%)	56 (81.2%)	0.7
1–80 g/week	8 (17.4%)	38 (82.6%)	
Over 80 g/week	15 (23.4%)	49 (76.6%)	
Atherogenic			
<5 (low risk)	22 (16.8%)	109 (83.2%)	0.04*
>5 (high risk)	14 (31.1%)	31 (68.9%)	
Diabetes			
No	13 (21.7%)	47 (78.3%)	0.7
Yes	23 (19.3%)	96 (80.7%)	
Hypertension			
No	16 (21.1%)	60 (78.9%)	0.8
Yes	20 (19.4%)	83 (80.6%)	
Dyslipidemia			
No	20 (18.7%)	87 (81.3%)	0.6
Yes	16 (22.2%)	56 (77.6%)	

Variables	Absence ED	Presence ED	p
Diabetes drugs			
Can produce ED	8 (14.5%)	47 (85.5%)	0.22
No produce ED	15 (23.4%)	49 (76.6%)	
Hypertension drugs			
Can produce ED	16 (19.8%)	65 (80.2%)	0.85
No produce ED	3 (21.4%)	11 (78.6%)	

*p < 0.05: statistically significant.

Table 2. Description of qualitative variables in relation to the main variable: ED (presence or absence) in the sample surveyed.

2. Variables analysis

- Age.
- Level of education.
- Civil status.
- Height, weight and body mass index (BMI).
- SBP and DBP.
- Smoking habit, number of cigarettes/day, year smoking started, ex-smoker, year smoking stopped.
- Alcohol consumption, grams alcohol/week.
- Consumption of other drugs, frequency and type.
- Blood test: glucose, glycated haemoglobin, total cholesterol, LDL cholesterol, HDL cholesterol, triglycerides, atherogenic index, creatinine, urea, GOT, GPT, gamma-GT and PSA.
- Urine test: microalbuminuria, proteinuria and creatinine clearance.
- Electrocardiogram (ECG).
- Diabetes diagnosed at least 1 year ago and prescribed drugs to treat it.
- High blood pressure diagnosed at least 1 year ago and prescribed drugs to treat it.
- Dyslipidaemia (hypercholesterolemia) diagnosed at least 1 year ago and prescribed drugs to treat it.
- Concomitant diseases of at least 1 year and drugs (up to three).
- SHIM questionnaire and ED according to SHIM.

- LISAT-8 questionnaire set out per items:
- LISAT-8 Variable Test:

To all those surveyed, a quality-of-life test was provided, the LISAT-8. The Quality of Life Satisfaction questionnaire of Fugl-Meyer et al., or LISAT-8, is a list or inventory that assesses the satisfaction of the life of the adult population undergoing rehabilitation programmes, which have later been studied in ED patients. This list has been validated in several languages, including Spanish, in a masculine population with ED. This self-assessment questionnaire contains eight items that score on a Likert-type scale [31–35]:

(1) Highly insatisfactory; (2) insatisfactory; (3) somewhat insatisfactory; (4) somewhat satisfactory; (5) satisfactory and (6) highly satisfactory, which measure satisfaction with eight different facets of the patient's life: life in general, sex life, relations with partner, family life, relations with friends and people known, entertainment, occupational situation and economic situation.

2.1. Statistical analysis

The qualitative variables are presented as the exact value and percentages, while the quantitative values are mean and standard deviation (SD).

Statistical comparison between means used the Student's *t* test for independent groups or the Mann-Whitney U test was used if normality conditions (using the Kolmogorov-Smirnoff or the Shapiro-Wilks test) were not fulfilled. A chi-squared test was done with the qualitative variables.

3. Results

Of the 210 people selected, 179 correctly completed the questionnaire, 85.2%. The mean age was 64.5 ± 11.6 years.

When analysing all study variables in relation to the main variable, presence or absence of ED, age was seen to play an important role as ED incidence increased with age to reach 95% in the 71–86 years age group as opposed to 5% when ED was absent. Blood pressure showed no significant relationship in connection with the studied variable, and the same holds for BMI and its subdivision into two ranges: normal weight and obese. Neither cigarette smoking nor alcohol consumption appeared to influence the presence of ED. Likewise, the sociological-type variables (civil status, level of education) presented no significant relationship.

With the biochemical variables collected from blood tests, we found a significant relationship with the atherogenic index and its variable recoded as a high and low atherogenic risk ($p < 0.04$). A mean of glycaemia of 126 mg/dl was obtained in the group in which ED was present, which is the cut-off point proposed by the ADA117 (American Diabetes Association) to consider a subject diabetic. Similarly, glycated haemoglobin showed data in the two groups, which could be considered an almost diabetic alteration to glucose metabolism.

In the hepatic profile, it is worth stressing that GPT transaminases and gamma GT showed a statistically significant relationship with ED presence. No significant results were obtained with the other parameters.

With the presence of diabetes, HBP and dyslipidaemia, this study revealed no significant relationship in relation to ED presence for each disease. However, a statistically significant association with these diseases was observed when CVR increased, according to the Framinghan

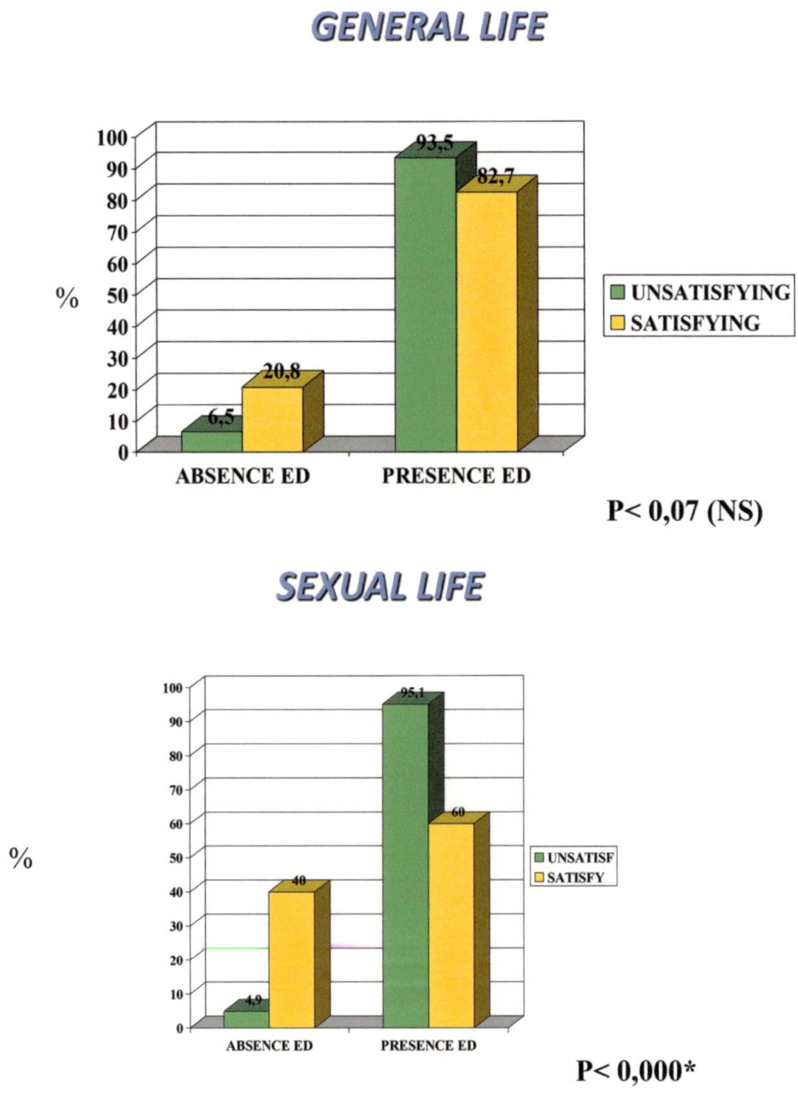

Graph 1. The LISAT-8 questionnaire results. **Sexual life, p < 0.00001 (statistically significant).**

tables (based on the study of Wilson et al. published in Circulation [61] (known as Framinghan study) to calculate the coronary risk in patients of our study).

Disease duration showed no such significant relationship, and the same holds for the drugs used to treat these three pathologies [37–39].

The coronary risk calculated according to the Framinghan tables obtained a statistically significant result, similarly to excess risk (the difference between coronary risk and the average risk assigned for each age) for the presence of ED.

No significant relationship was found for the diseases associated with these three pathologies ($p < 0.46$), but the drugs used for their treatment showed a relationship close to statistical significance ($p < 0.07$) [40–48].

In our study, the LISAT 8 test demonstrated that ED affected significantly health-associated quality of life, for two items, sex life and economic situation were statistically significant (see **Graph 1**), and the other general life and working life items tended to significance (see **Graph 2**). A significant relationship was also noted in the LISAT test score and was significantly lower among individuals with ED. Furthermore, a statistical relationship was seen when grouping the eight items into three dimensions or scales with love life and emotional life, a relationship close to significance was noted for those satisfied with the occupational life or the economic dimension, but no relationship was seen with the social life dimension [31–35].

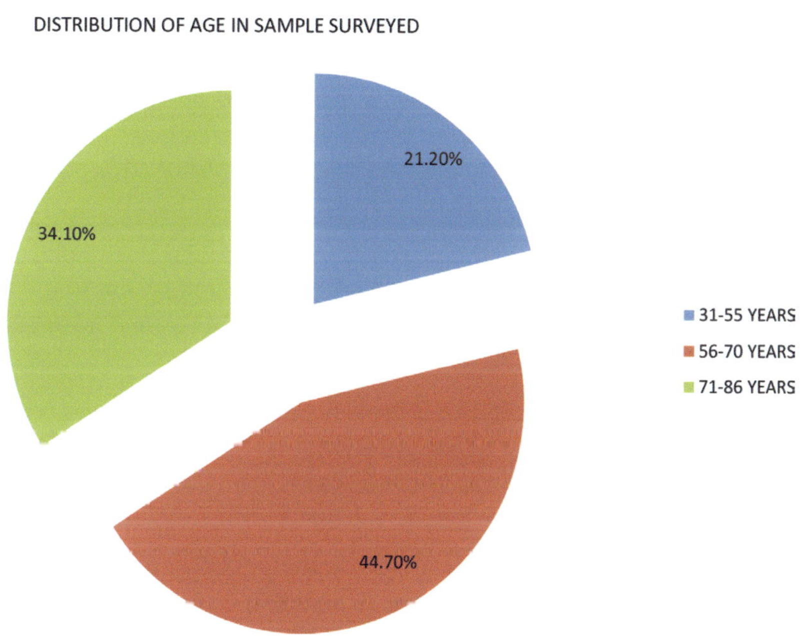

Graph 2. Distribution of age groups in the sample surveyed. **General life, $p < 0.007$ (not statistically significant).**

4. Discussion

Erectile dysfunction is defined as being unable to sufficiently obtain and maintain an erection to enjoy sexual satisfaction [1–6].

In the past, both physicians and the general population considered ED an inevitable consequence of age. Yet, our knowledge of masculine sexual function and dysfunction is increasing, and there is an important wide therapeutic range that needs to be explored. The World Health Organisation (WHO) has defined sexual health as a basic human right which includes the capacity to enjoy and control sexual behaviour, as a freedom that neither inhibits sexual responses nor is detrimental for sexual relations because of fear, shame, sense of guilt, false beliefs or other factors, and as a freedom so that organic diseases and other deficiencies do not interfere with either sexual or reproductive function. The WHO acknowledges ED as a health problem with the same degree of invalidity and severity as rheumatoid arthritis and heart angina [8–30].

Despite not being a pathology implying vital risk, ED greatly affects quality of life and could be a first sign of a serious underlying disease and is therefore of interest in patients who come to primary health care (PHC) consultations for this pathology [31–35].

Erectile dysfunction is a health problem and, unlike the traditional concept of it being merely a consequence of ageing, today it is considered a highly prevalent pathology. Apart from psychological factors to which much importance was attached in the 1950–1970s, the organic causes in the population assessed by the PHC are particularly interesting. Indeed in the NIH's consensus conference in 1993, it was assumed that most organic ED cases are associated with vascular risk factors: diabetes, hypercholesterolaemia, hypertension and smoking [9–17].

Atherosclerosis is the cause of 40% of ED cases in men aged over 50. Moreover, it damages endothelium and smooth muscle of the sinusoids of cavernous bodies, which makes the relaxation of arteries and smooth sinusoidal muscle in men difficult. This poor relaxation of smooth muscle in men is the most important pathogenic factor of ED [3].

Cardiac ischaemia, HBP, diabetes mellitus (DM), hyperlipidaemia, and smoking are pathological processes, which are indirectly associated with ED given their implication in the formation of atherosclerotic plates. Increased total cholesterol or LDL-c and lowered HDL-c are associated with arterial failure [37–40].

The relationship between ED and HBP is clearly well-established, which was confirmed by a study of Cuellar et al., who found a 46.5% prevalence for ED in patients with HBP. This high prevalence of ED in hypertensive patients can be basically due to two reasons: the lesions that HBP causes in arteries and the endothelium of cavernous bodies, and the effects on erections that anti-hypertensives may bring about [48–54].

As regards DM, ED prevalence varies between 20 and 50%. In Spain, a recent study places prevalence at 15.6% for diabetics type 1 and at 29.6% for diabetics type 2. The appearance of ED tends to take place before 10 years have elapsed since diagnosing DM. The occurrence of ED is between 10 and 15 years earlier among diabetics than in the general population; 12% of patients have ED as their first symptom of diabetes. Studies done in Italy and Spain have demonstrated that ED in patients with DM type 2 can be an indicator of a silent ischaemic cardiopathy [44–47].

ED presence in our study is associated with a significant index of patients with high CVR, which is substantially higher than that considered in other works which also include patients without CVRF. In relation to other studies, the differences in prevalence found could be due to these studies also including patients with no CVR.

In our study, we have been able to verify how vascular risk factors show high prevalence; we can observe how the mean figures for both glycaemia and glycated haemoglobin are clearly pathologic, and how 80.7% of diabetics present ED (See **Graph 3**). The HBP figures also reveal that hypertensive patients present 80.6% of ED (see **Graph 4**). Moreover, 77.6% of patients

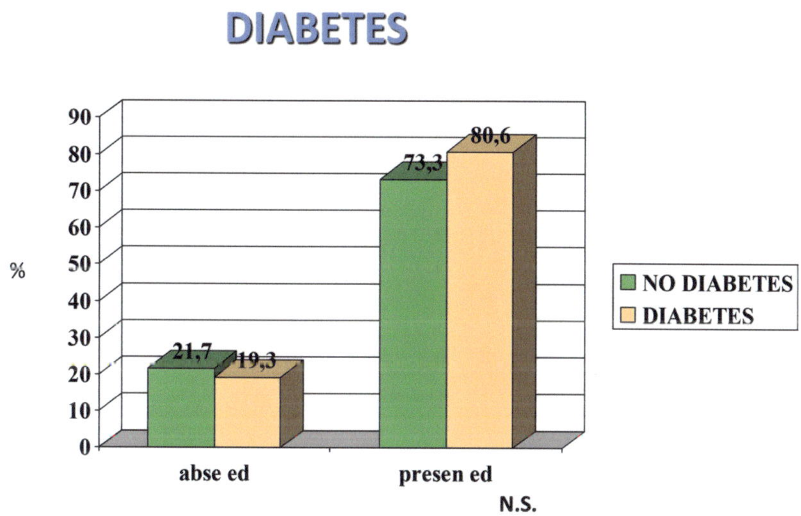

Graph 3. Diabetes%. N.S.

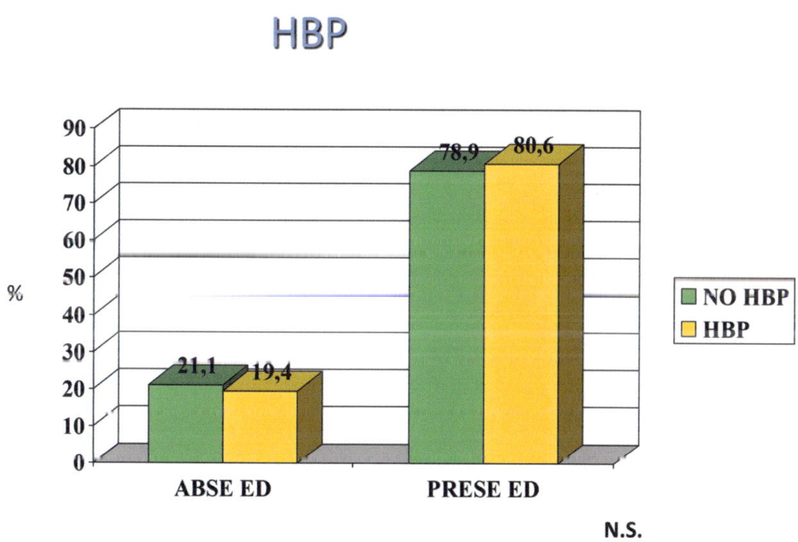

Graph 4. HBP%. N.S.

with dyslipidaemia show ED as opposed to 22.4% who do not. Our study also reveals that 72.7% of those who report smoking daily have ED.

Using the atherogenic index and CVR, and according to the Framinghan tables, the overall assessment indicates a highly significant relationship with ED [36–42] (see **Graph 5**).

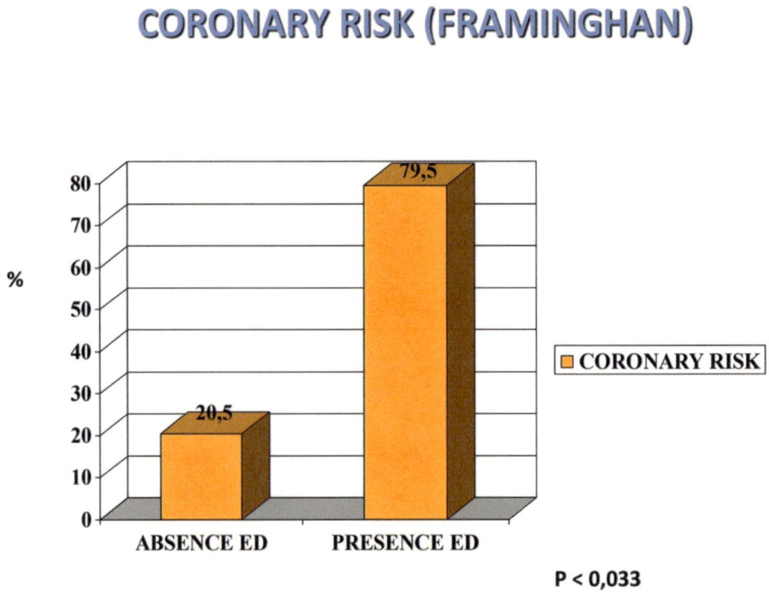

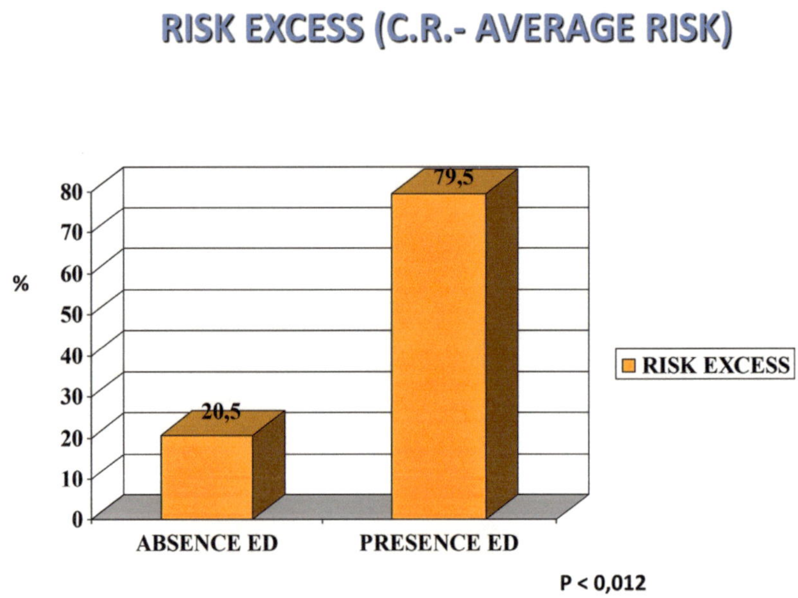

Graph 5. Coronary risk (Framinghan) %, $p < 0.033$.

It is worthwhile highlighting the consumption of drugs related with ED as none of them actually mention this side effect in their technical information, and many others do not consider it either. It is assumed that beta-blockers cause ED, but the effect of beta-adrenergics is rarely evaluated (or they are thought to not cause erectile alterations), yet terbutaline and salbutamol (greatly consumed in our sample) are indicated treatments in priapism with a subsequent effect on ED. This study shows a tendency to statistical significance between the consumption of certain drugs to treat associated diseases and ED, which confirms the suspicions of the relationship between these drugs and ED [41–45, 54–60].

From our study, the following conclusions may be drawn:

1. There is a high prevalence of erectile dysfunction in patients with high cardiovascular risk.
2. Advanced age is a risk factor for erectile dysfunction.
3. Erectile dysfunction improves if cardiovascular risk factors are better controlled.
4. Our patients' pluripathology status implies aggressive polymedication, which the doctor must consider as it increases the risk of erectile dysfunction.
5. Erectile dysfunction has a negative effect on quality of life and especially affects physical aspects, love life and life with a partner.

Author details

Ángel Celada Rodríguez[1], Pedro Juan Tárraga López[1]*, José Antonio Rodríguez Montes[2], Mª Loreto Tarraga Marcos[1] and Carmen Celada Roldan[3]

*Address all correspondence to: pedrojuan.tarraga@uclm.es

1 University of Castilla la Mancha, Albacete, Spain

2 Autonomous University of Madrid, Madrid, Spain

3 UDMPF Cartagena Mar Menor, Murcia, Spain

References

[1] Más García M. Aspectos actuales de la fisiopatología de la erección. En Arrondo Arrondo JL, editor. Actualización en Andrologia. Servicio Navarro de Salud; 1999. pp. 216-222

[2] Más García M. Bases Fisiológicas de la sexualidad. Respuesta sexual. En: Castelo-Branco C, editor. Sexualidad Humana. Una aproximación integral. Madrid. Panamericana; 2005. pp. 28-30

[3] Burnett A. Role of nitric oxide in physiology of erection. Biology of Reproduction. 1995;**52**:485-489

[4] Moreira Machado A. Etiopatogenia de la Disfunción eréctil. En: Arrondo Arrondo JL, editor. Actualización en Andrología. Servicio Navarro de Salud; 1999. pp. 224-239

[5] Feldman HA, Goldestein I, Hatzichristou DG, Krane RJ, McKinlay JB. Impotence and its medical and psychological correlates: Results of the Massachusetts Male Aging Study. Journal of Urology. 1994;**151**:54-61

[6] Martin Morales A, Sánchez Cruz JJ, Saenz de Tejada I, Rodríguez Vela L, Jiménez-Cruz JF, Burgos-Rodríguez R. Prevalence and independent risk factors for erectile dysfunction in Spain: Results of the Epidemiología de la Disfunción Eréctil Masculina Study. Journal of Urology. 2001;**166**:569-575

[7] Guirao Sánchez L, García-Giralda Ruiz L, Sandoval Martínez C, Mocciaro Loveccio A. Disfunción eréctil en atención primaria como marcador del estado de salud: factores asociados y respuesta al sildenafilo. Aten Primaria. 2002;**30**:290-296

[8] Pomerol Monseny JM. Principios básicos en el diagnóstico de la disfunción eréctil. En: Arrondo Arrondo JL, editor. Actualización en Andrología. Servicio Navarro de Salud; 1999. pp. 259-265

[9] Gades NM, Nehra A, Jacobson DJ, McGree ME, Ghirman CJ, Rhodes T, Roberts RO, Liebre MM, Jacobsen SJ. Association between smoking and erectile dysfunction: A population-based study. American Journal of Epidemiology. 2005;**161**:346-351

[10] Rodríguez Vela L. Impotencia e hipertensión arterial. Medicina Clínica (Barc). 2002;**119**: 534-536

[11] Cuéllar de León AJ, Ruíz García V, Campos González JC, Pérez Hoyos S, Brotons Multó F. Prevalencia de la disfunción eréctil en pacientes con hipertensión arterial. Medicina Clínica (Barc). 2002;**119**:521-526

[12] Burchardt M, Burchardt T, Baer L, Kiss AJ, Pawar RV, Shabsigh A, et al. Hipertensión is associated with severe erectile dysfunction. Journal of Urology. 2000;**164**:1188-1191

[13] Enzlin P, Chantal M, Van Der Cruel A, Vanderschueren V, Demyttenaere K. Prevalence and predictors of sexual dysfunction in patients with type 1 diabetes. Diabetes Care. 2003;**26**:409-414

[14] Romeo JH, Seftel AD, Madhun ZT, Aron DC. Sexual function in men with diabetes type 2: Association with glycemic control. Journal of Urology. 2000;**163**:788-791

[15] Ming W, Macera CA, Davis DR, Hornung CA, Nankin HA, Blair SN. Total cholesterol and high density lipoprotein cholesterol as important predictors of erectile dysfunction. American Journal of Epidemiology. 1994;**140**:930-932

[16] Van Steenbergen W. Alcohol, liver cirrhosis and disorders in sex hormone metabolisme. Acta Clinica Belgica. 1993;**48**:269-283

[17] Fuster Bellido T, Martínez Ques D, Faus Mascarell E, Colominas Sarrió P, Plá Vallá R, Arlandis Puig A. Disfunción eréctil. Prevalencia y factores de riesgo asociados. Sexología Integral. 2006;**3**:210-212

[18] Cruz Navarro N. Alternativas actuales en la terapia oral de la Disfunción Eréctil. En Arrondo Arrondo JL, editor. Actualización en Andrología. Servicio Navarro de Salud; 1999. pp. 266-286

[19] Buvat J, Buvaut-Herbaut M, Lemaire A, et al. Les traitements médicaux de l'impuissance. En Arvis G, editor. Andrologie. Paris: Maloine Ed; 1991. pp. 2015-2038

[20] Krane RJ, Goldstein I, Sáenz de Tejada I. Medical progress: Impotence. New England Journal of Medicine. 1989;**321**:1648-1659

[21] Goldstein I, Lue TF, Padma-Nathan H, et al. Oral sildenafil in the treatment of erectile dysfunction. New England Journal of Medicine. 1998;**338**:1397-1404

[22] Cuzin B, Emrich HM, Meuleman EJH, et al. Sildenafil: A 6-month, double-blind, placebo-controlled, flexible dose-escalation study in patients with erectile dysfunction. International Journal of Impotence Research. 1998;**10**:S1-S3

[23] Stief y cols. Eficacia mantenida y tolerabilidad de vardenafilo a lo largo de 2 años de tratamiento en varones con disfunción eréctil. International Journal of Clinical Practice. 2004;**58**:320-329

[24] Montorsi F, McDermott TE, Morgan R, et al. Efficacy and safety of fixed-dose oral sildenafil in the treatment of erectile dysfunction of various etiologies. Urology. 1999;**53**:1011-1018

[25] Morales A, Gingell C, Collins M, et al. Clinical safety of oral sildenafil citrate in the treatment of erectile dysfunction. International Journal of Impotence Research. 1998;**10**:69-74

[26] Brindley GS. Cavernosal alpha blockade: A new technique for investigation and treating erectile impotence. British Journal of Psychiatry. 1983;**143**:322

[27] Bennet AH, Carpenter AJ, Barada JH. An improved vasoactive drug combination for a pharmacological erection program. Journal of Urology. 1991;**146**:1564-1565

[28] Saénz de Tejada I, Moncada I. Inyección intracavernosa de vasodilatadores para el tratamiento de la impotencia. En: Saénz de Tejada I, Allona A, editors. Erección, eyaculación y sus trastornos. Madrid: Fomento Salud; 1997. p. 323

[29] Roselló Barbará M. Tratamiento quirúrgico de la Disfunción Eréctil. Prótesis de pene. En: Arrondo Arrondo JL, editor. Actualización en Andrología. Servicio Navarro de Salud; 1999. p. 308

[30] Rosen RC, Cappelleri JC, Smith MD, Lipsky J, Pena BM. Development and evaluation of an abridged, 5-item version of the International Index of Erectile Function (IIEF-5) as a diagnostic tool for erectile dysfunction. International Journal of Impotence Research. 1999;**11**:319-326

[31] Fugl-Meyer AR, Bräholm IB, Fugl-Meyer KS. Happiness and domain-specific life satisfaction in adult northern Swedes. Clinical Rehabilitation. 1991;**5**:25-33

[32] Fugl-Meyer AR, Lodner G, Bräholm IB, Fugl-Meyer KS. On life satisfaction in male erectile dysfunction. International Journal of Impotence Research. 1997;**9**:141-148

[33] Conway K, Chaput M, Fugl-Meyer KS, Fugl-Meyer A, Kubin M. Linguistic validation of the Fugl-Meyer Life Satisfaction Checklist (LISAT). 7th Annual Conference of the International Society of Quality of Life. Vancouver 2000. Quality of Life Research. 2000;**9**(Abstract P-41):319

[34] Rejas J, Gil de Miguel A, San Isidro C, Palacios G, Carrasco P. Adaptación cultural y validación psicométrica del cuestionario de satisfacción con la vida de Fugl-Meyer-LISAT 8 en población española masculina con disfunción eréctil. Pharmaeconomics Sp Res Art. 2004

[35] Rejas Gutiérrez J, Gil de Miguel A, Martínez Sánchez EM, Díaz García E. Construcción de una variable subrogada de detección de disfunción eréctil a partir de la versión española de Cuestionario de satisfacción cn la vida "LISAT 8". Semergen. 2005;**31**:462-470

[36] Artigao Rodenas LM. Prevalencia de factores de riesgo cardiovascular en la provincia de Albacete [Tesis Doctoral]. Universidad Autónoma de Madrid; 1997. 125-155

[37] Díaz Díaz JL, Argüeso Armesto RM. Actitud ante pacientes con dislipemia. En: Guías Clínicas de la Sociedad Gallega de Medicina Interna. 2006

[38] Castelli WP. Lipids, risk factors and ischaemic heart disease. Atherosclerosis. 1996;**124**:S1-S9

[39] National Cholesterol Education Program. Executive summary of the tird report of the national cholesterol education program (NCEP) expert panel on detection, evaluation, and treatment of high blood cholesterol in adults (Adult Treatment Panel III). Journal of the American Medical Association. 2001;**285**:2486-2497

[40] Villamil Cajoto I, Díaz Peromingo JA, Sánchez Leira J, García Suárez F, Saborido Forjan J, Iglesias Gallego M. Disfunción eréctil: un problema poco valorado en Medicina Interna. Estudio de pacientes y medicación relacionada. An Med Inter (Madrid). 2006;**23**:115-118

[41] Drugs that cause sexual dysfunction: An update. Medical Letter. 1992;**34**:73-78

[42] Brock GB, Lue TF. Drug-induced male sexual dysfunction. An update. Drug Safety. 1993;**8**: 414-426

[43] Finger WW, Luna M, Slagle MA. Medications that may contribute to sexual disorders: A guide to assessment and treatment in family practice. The Journal of Family Practice. 1997;**44**:33-43

[44] Lipshultz LL, Kim ED. Treatment of erectile dysfunction in men with diabetes. Journal of the American Medical Association. 1999;**281**:465-466

[45] Rivero M. "Drogas y fármacos erectolíticos". En: III Curso de farmacología del músculo liso urinario & genital masculino. Bajado de Internet (www.uro.org.ar) el 13/02/2007

[46] Davis SN, Granner DK. Insulina, Hipoglucemiantes orales y propiedades farmacológicas del páncreas endocrino, en Goodman & Gilman "Bases farmacológicas de la terapéutica". 10ª edición. México: McGraw Hill; 2003. pp. 1720-1725

[47] Lebovitz HE. Secretagogos de insulina. En: Le Roith D, Taylor SI, Olefsky JM, editors. Diabetes Mellitus. Fundamentos y Clínica. 2ª edición. México: Mcgraw Hill; 2003. pp. 960-970

[48] Foyt HL, Ghazzi MN, Hanley RM, et al. Tiazolidindionas. en: Le Roith D, Taylor SI, Olefsky JM, editors. Diabetes Mellitus. Fundamentos y clínica. 2ª edición. México: McGraw Hill; 2ª edición2003. pp. 982-992

[49] Llisterri Caro JL, Sánchez Sánchez F, Brotons Muntó F. Disfunción sexual en la hipertensión arterial. Hipertensión. 2005;**22**:59-72

[50] Cuellar de León AJ, Campos González JC, Brotons Muntó F, et al. Hipertensión arterial y disfunción eréctil. Grupo de Urología de la SVMFYC; 2005

[51] Jackson G, Betteridge J, Dean J, et al. A systematic approach to erectile dysfunction in the cardiovascular patient: A consensus statement. International Journal of Clinical Practice. 1999;**53**:445-451

[52] Grimm RH, Grandits G, Svendsen K, et al. Sexual problems and antihypertensive drugs treatment: Results of the Treatment of Mild Hipertensión Study (THOMS). Journal of Urology. 1996;**155**:634-644

[53] Grimm R, Grandits G, Prineas R, et al. Long-term effects on sexual function of five antihypertensive drugs and nutritional hygienic treatment in hypertensive men and women. Hypertension. 1997;**29**:8-14

[54] Wassertheil-Smoller S, Blaufox MD, Oberman A, et al. Effect of antihypertensive on sexual function and quality of life. The TAIM Study. Annals of Internal Medicine. 1991;**114**:613-620

[55] Montejo Al, Llorca G, Izquierdo JA, et al. Incidence of sexual dysfunction associated to different antidepressant agents. A 5-year prospective and multicentre study in 1022 patients. The Journal of Clinical Psychiatry. 2001;**62**:10-21

[56] Cappelleri JC, Rosen RC, Smith MD, et al. Diagnostic evaluation of the erectile function domain of the International Index of Erectile Function. Urology. 1995;**54**:346-351

[57] Rosen RC, Riley A, Wagner G, et al. The International Index of Erectile Function (IIEF): A multidimensional scale for assessment of erectile dysfunction. Urology. 1997;**49**:822-830

[58] Bataller i Perelló V. Problemas y síntomas sexuales del varón. Sexología Integral. 2007;**4**: 49-50

[59] Muller SC, El-Damanhoury H, Ruth J. Hypertension and impotence. European Urology. 1991;**19**:29-34

[60] Sánchez Cruz JJ, Cabrera León A, Martín Morales A, et al. Male erectile dysfunction and health-related quality of life. European Urology. 2003;**44**:245-253

[61] Wilson PWF, D'Agostino RB, Levy D, et al. Prediction of coronary heart disease using risk factor categories. Circulation. 1998;**97**:1837-1847

Section 3

Hypogonadism

Chapter 3

Hypogonadism in Male Sexual Dysfunction

Dana Stoian, Ioana Mozos, Marius Craina,
Corina Paul, Iulian Velea, Adalbert Schiller and
Mihaela Craciunescu

Additional information is available at the end of the chapter

http://dx.doi.org/10.5772/intechopen.69107

Abstract

Normal testosterone level is influencing all the steps of the male psychosexual development: intrauterine neonatal and final psychosexual development.. At pubertal stage, the quality of testosterone secretion is conditioning the development of the mature male phenotype. In adult life, eugonadism sustains desire, arousal, determines spontaneous erections, facilitates stimulated erection, influencing the response rate to medication. Moreover, eugonadism sustain daydreaming and phantasies, both needed for a normal sexual life. The pathogenic mechanism of all these actions is presented. Talking about hypogonadism means not only the classical types of hypogonadism: due to classical testicular disease of central, hypothalamic and hypophysis disease, but also the partial testosterone deficiency induces by aging (late onset hypogonadism), weight increase (up to 30% of males with metabolic syndrome and 50% of males with diabetes) or secondary hypogonadism described in chronic use of steroids or after long exposure to stress, especially in young males. All these types of hypogonadism, that affect young, middle aged or old males will be presented separately. A therapeutic approach that is individualized for each type of hypogonadism, should consider positive and possible negative effects and all alternatives will be presented: life style changes, sustained weight loss, increase exercise, supplemental therapy, pro fertility treatment.

Keywords: male sexual function, hypogonadism, late-onset hypogonadism, testosterone, supplemental treatment

1. Introduction

Testosterone is an essential hormone that influences part of sexual function in males.

Androgens directly influence the formation of male genital structures as an active process, start in the intrauterine life, sustain the phenotypic complete adult male pattern during development in puberty, and maintain the male phenotype during the entire life. Also androgens, together with other sexual steroids, do regulate sexual behavior, testosterone being the principal determinant of the sex drive not only in males but also in females. Male sexual response involves the presence of erection, a phenomenon influenced/sustained and modulated by testosterone levels. In these cases, the response rate to treatment is also dependent on the intratesticular testosterone. Psychosexual development is also conditioned by testosterone presence during childhood and puberty. Testosterone deficiency, regardless of inherited diseases, iatrogenic causes, metabolic disease or acquired causes, will impair normal sexual life and will condition the response to hormonal and non-hormonal treatment. Testosterone deficiency should be considered not only in the classical hypogonadism cases, with central or peripheral forms of disease, but also in the more frequent cause of subclinical, late onset of disease that affects half of the diabetic population, 30% of the metabolic syndrome male population and some of the elderly male population.

2. Role of testosterone in sexual function in males

Normal sexuality in both male and women presumes a normal phenotypic structure, sexual identity development and sexual orientation. Especially in males, testosterone influences all aspects of normal sexual function. In order to develop a normal sexual response, we need complete, congruent or not, sexual structures, sexual development and psychosexual components.

2.1. Testosterone effects in male sexualization: organic aspects

After the fertilization of the egg, the chromosomal sex is formed. According to the karyoptype [1], there are two ways of evolution:

The active way: In the presence of the sexual active chromosome Y, mainly the SRY gene, located on the short arm, favors the preprogrammed male gonadic development. The expression of SRY induces the organization of indifferent gonads to Sertoli cell differentiation [2], Antimullerian hormone production (AMH) [3], and secondary to testosterone synthesis from the Leydig cells [4]. The androgen presence will generate the evolution of Wolff tract structure (paracrine effect on the homonymous site) masculinization of the external genitals (weeks 12–16) and involution of Muller tract structures. Notably, testosterone in order to be active at the external genital ridge has to be converted to 5 α-dihydrotestosterone. Also, the testicular descent from the abdominal cavity is a dihydrotestosterone-dependent phenomenon. Normal testosterone levels, normal enzymatic apparatus and also normal testosterone receptor activity are needed to obtain the physiological effects.

The passive way: Feminization appears only in the absence of active Y chromosome expressing SRY gene, when regardless of the karyotype (46XX, 46 XY, 45X, 45 XX/45 XY), their evolution follows the free, automatic female gonad development, that only starts after the 3rd month of intra-gestational development [5]. In the absence of testosterone, there is an involution of the Wolff tract structures with a spontaneous, preprogramed differentiation of Muller tract structures: fallopian tubes, uterus and superior one-third of the vagina. **Figure 1** summarizes the intrauterine changes in the genital area in both the sexes.

We can consider that the steroids have a major function in somatosexual development: organizational function—in the development phases, causing permanent changes in the body but also in the brain, and an activational function, active later in life, which will guide behavior.

The dismorphic brain changes are described by numerous studies. Testosterone is considered to be anxiolytic, anti-depressant and facilitates spatial abilities [6].

The postnatal somatosexual differentiation comprises small changes during early childhood. There are minimal somatic differences between sexes, steroid-independent: more female sex babies, boys are lesser maturated compared to girls, growth increase sooner in girls than boys, with increased size of extremities, increased mandibula, flattening of the trunk with important changes in cognition [7].

The puberty period represents the major second transformation period, both in genital and in nongenital spheres [8]. Secondary to the hypothalamus-hypophysis axis disinhibition,

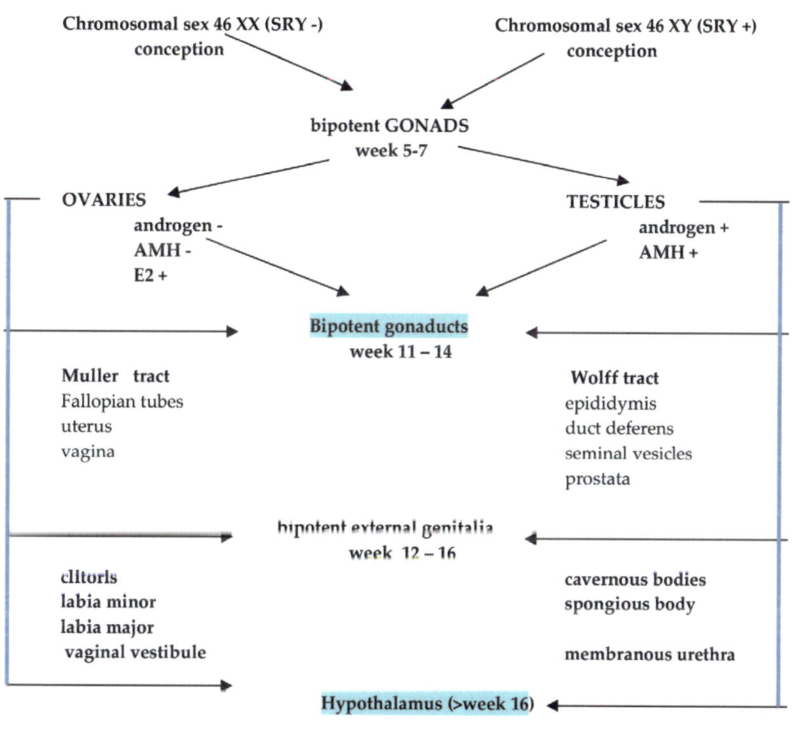

Figure 1. Scheme of the somatosexual differentiation in the intrauterine period.

between 8 and 13 years of age in females and 9–13.5 years of age in boys, the production of sexual steroids increases dramatically and significant bodily changes appear secondary to exposure to sexual steroids. The somatic changes are measurable by the Tanner stage evaluation of secondary sexual characters (breast and pubic hair development in girls, external genitals and pubic hair in boys). In males, the following changes are described, all androgen dependent [9]: testosterone-dependent effects are increase in muscular mass, bone growth, growth of larynx and deepening of voice, inhibition of breast development, stimulation of spermatogenesis, whereas the dihydrotestosterone-dependent effects are phallic growth, development of pubic hair, and activity of sebaceous glands.

Table 1 summarizes the somatic changes observed in puberty, with the onset timing.

At the end of puberty, we have clear somatic differences between males and females, all sexual steroid-dependent [8, 9]. Notably, the full male pattern is present at the end of puberty, but the complete emotional evolution is not yet present. This is a high-risk period for sexual experiences.

During adulthood, eugonadism is important to maintain and sustain the previous organic changes. It has only a permissive role for maintaining normal sexual responses.

Regardless of diseases, aging is associated with physiological hormonal changes. There are several studies [10–12] suggesting that aging is one of the major factors involved in sexual

Male gender	Mean age (years)
Increase penis length	11–12
Increase testes volume	
Acne	12
Prostate growth	12.5
Pubarche (P2)	12–13
Growth spurt	12–13
Sesamoid bone	13
Accelerate increase in penis diameter	13–14
Axillary hair (AH1)	14–15
Pubarche (P4)	14.5
Voice change	14–15
Facial hair	14–15
Pubarche (P5)	15–16
Complete spermatogenesis	16
Epiphyseal plate closure	>17

Table 1. Somatic changes in male puberty.

functional changes in males. There is physiological involution of all endocrine glands, with decreases in thyroid, adrenal and gonadal hormone production [12].

Many epidemiological studies describe a physiological decrease in total and free testosterone levels [13–15]. Many changes are described with important sexual symptoms, similar to the presence of overt hypogonadism, with important diseases linked to this testosterone deficiency: bone demineralization [16], increased cardiovascular risk [17], frailty [18], weight gain [19], dyslipidemia [20] and increased general mortality [21–23].

2.2. Testosterone role in male sexuality: psychosexual aspects

The psychosexual development is conditioned from the beginning in neonatal life.

Psychosexual differentiation refers to gender identity, respectively, self-identification as male or female, gender role, comprising different behavior in males and females, gender orientation, representing the choice of sexual partner, respectively cognitive differences [24]. Classically, gender identity was considered imprinted postnatally only by social attitudes, words, family dynamics, comparison of own body to pears, cultural differences, degree of exposure to nakedness [24], learning theory (gender identity is shaped by personal models and cultural influences, according to the interaction with parents), cognitive development theory (observation and imitation of behaviors appropriate for each gender), and biosocial interaction (society norms influencing subsequent behavior patterns in the childhood) [24].

Testosterone influences cell survival, anatomical connections and neurochemical activity, being responsible for brain differences in structure and function [25]. It is known that prenatal androgen exposure influences children's sex-typed play behavior [26]. Genetic diseases with abnormal sexual steroid hormones can be used in the evaluation of sexual steroid impact on sexual identity: exposure to androgenic progestins increases male-typical behavior [27], and exposure to antiandrogenic products will decrease female-typical behaviors [28, 29]. There is a correlation between testosterone levels in maternal blood and amniotic fluid and sex-type behavior in childhood [30, 31]. Also, the new explanation for the "toy theory" is that androgen exposure favors interest for space movements, by influencing the development of visual fields [32, 33].

There is clear evidence that testosterone and dihydrotestosterone exposure can influence gender identity [33, 34]. Androgens have a facilitating and not a determinant role in gender identity development [35].

During childhood, psychosexual development is mainly socially dependent and not steroid-dependent: starting at approximately 1 year of age, boys and girls are aware of gender differences at an age of 2–3 years of their own gender, at 3 years of the behavior that belongs to the gender role, and from age 5 they play with the same gender peers. Before the age of 6 "sexual—genital" behaviors are reported but have no conscious significance, being just a pleasure action. After the age of 6 years, these behaviors are stable due to the juvenile pause. The development is free of androgen influence, due to the gonadostat inhibition, that stays till the spontaneous disinhibition of gonadotropic-gonadal axis. Still indirect effects are seen.

Puberty is a period with important changes in psychosexual behavior. In early adolescence, exposure to increased testosterone levels in boys will induce increased aggression and social dominance [36], whereas premature estrogen exposure in girls will favor mood changes [37]. During puberty, steroid hormones-related changes in the frontal lobe are different in boys and girls, favoring phonological skills in women and special skills in boys [38].

The hormonal and physical changes that occur during puberty also contribute in indirect ways to differences between adolescent boys and adolescent girls. In girls, secondary sexual changes will induce social reactions from peers, parents, teachers, and friends. Adolescence is associated with changing social roles, and there is good reason to believe that gender socialization intensifies at that time of life [39, 40].

During adolescence typical sexual behaviors will appear: in early adolescence physical changes dominate, with insecurity, sexual curiosity and exploration. Auto stimulation is reactivated, typical sexual in this case, different from the unconscious stimulation in the early childhood period. Androgens are the most important hormones that induce sexual drive [41]. Monogamously focused relationships, growing maturity, and responsibility characterize middle adolescence, and late adolescence is the period of beginning of mature sexuality and accumulation of sexual skills.

The relationship between testosterone and sexual behavior is more complex in humans than in animals, where sexual receptivity of the female and sexual interest in males is steroid-dependent [42]. In humans, there is a complex interference between genetic, hormonal, cultural, social, moral, and environmental influences.

In adults, testosterone sustains secondary sexual characters that were previously formed during puberty and directly influences all levels of sexual behavior:

Sexual fantasies are linked to testosterone levels, with a bimodal relationship, testosterone favors phantasies, and phantasies affect the testosterone levels [43]. Low testosterone levels in adult males change sexual interest even at the level of sexual fantasies [44, 45]. Even daydreaming is modulated by normal testosterone levels [45, 46].

Autostimulation and sexual actions are active behaviors, dependent on testosterone levels. The best evaluation of testosterone's involvement in these behaviors is represented by different hypogonadism males, due to different causes [47, 48]. Autostimulation is considered a testosterone-dependent behavior; some hypogonadism questionnaires (ANDROTEST) consider impaired masturbation as a positive criterium for hypogonadism [49].

2.3. Testosterone implication in male sexual responses

The classic male sexual response as described by Masters' and Johnson' comprises the following event succession: excitement, plateau, orgasm, and resolution [42] corresponding to different levels of arousal.

The most important sign of excitement is the appearance of erection. There are three types of erections.

2.3.1. Erection

Stimulated erection is the most complicated and sensitive type of erection, appearing triggered by voluntary actions (kissing, touching, reading, seeing, and smelling), verbal or non-verbal message, anyhow after an interaction with a partner, appearing within few seconds after correct sexual stimulation, regardless of the type of stimulation. After stimulation, the brain releases stimulatory neurotransmitters (dopamine, nitric oxide, oxytocin, serotonin), from oxytoninergic, serotonergic, and dopaminergic neurons located in "erection centers" in the limbic system (paraventricular and supraoptic nuclei) that will generate proerectile impulses via the parasympathetic system [50–53]. Parasympathetic impulses stimulate the spinal parasympathetic reflexogenic erection centers located at level S2–S4 [50] that will directly induce the vascular changes in the cavernous bodies, dilatation of arterioles, increased blow flow, decreased venous outflow due to compression of the subtunical venular plexuses, increase in oxygen pressure raising the penis, with subsidiary contraction of the ischiocavernosus muscles.

Testosterone influences erection both at central and at peripheral levels.

At CNS level, testosterone stimulates the synthesis, storage and release of proerectile neurotransmitters: dopamine, nitric oxide, and oxytocin [54–56].

At spinal level, the somatic innervation (motoneurons) of bulbo- and ischiocavernous muscles is testosterone-dependent, meaning that testosterone influences both the rigidity of the erection and the orgasmic capacity [57, 58].

At the corpus cavernous level, testosterone influences parasympathetic nerves that generate oxid nitric, facilitating NO secretion [59]. Testosterone also influences the quality of cavernous muscle relaxation, influencing the expression of alpha adrenoreceptors [60, 61]. Also, androgen deprivation favors cavernous muscle smooth cells apoptosis [62].

Testosterone and its metabolites at both central and peripheral neural pathways are crucial for maintaining and restoring erectile capacity. The mechanism of enhanced erection with testosterone depends not only on the peripheral neural pathway but also on the central neural pathway.

- Spontaneous erections are automatic, not controlled by a specific emotional content or response, being purely androgen-dependent. The mechanism of this erection is incompletely understood, but androgens play an important role [63, 64]. The role of this autonomous erection is nutritive for maintaining regular blood flow and oxygenation of the penis. Testosterone deficiency, depression, sleep apnea and altered REM phase sleep will impair this type of erection [65]. This type of erection is a very important diagnostic tool in the evaluation of erectile dysfunction and differentiation of organic from psychogenic erections.
- Mechanical erection is the most "independent" type of erection to testosterone level. The somatic pathway is active in cases of stimulated central erections, but also independent, in local mechanical stimulation. Testosterone is indirectly influencing this type of erection only by changing the properties of the cavernous smooth muscle units.

Desire is not present in the classical male sexual response but still is a very important step in male sexuality. Desire is considered to consist of a drive—biological component, cultural component (wish) and motivational component (individual and relational psychology) [66]. Testosterone and other androgens sustain the drive component [67].

3. Testosterone deficiency

In all cases of hypogonadism, major sexual symptoms are described [68–70]:

- Alteration of sexual desire and arousal with a significant decrease in frequency of sexual activity
- Decrease/altered quality of spontaneous erections
- Partial alteration of psychic erections: decrease in frequency, amplitude, and rigidity
- Alteration of orgasm and ejaculation proprieties
- Altered response to phosphodiesterase-5 inhibitors

The implication of testosterone deficiency is clear, but the level of deficiency where symptoms appear is still debatable. Effects of testosterone on sexual function are dose-dependent up to a level close to the lower limit of normal range. From this threshold level, the effects are maximal. In cases with testosterone levels very close to this limit, the benefits of testosterone replacement are minimal. Below the threshold, the sexual function is impaired [67]. Different thresholds are described according to the wanted effect of testosterone [71]. Also the threshold value is variable and may increase with aging concerning sexual function, higher testosterone levels are needed with aging for the same result [72], with possible individual values, according to personal sensitivity [73]. The prevalence of sexual symptoms increases as testosterone levels decrease: low libido and vigor for values lower than 15 nmol/L (4.3 ng/mL), disturbed sleep at values less than 10 nmol/L, neurovegetative symptoms and erectile dysfunction at values less than 8 nmol/L (2.3 ng/mL) [71] and 1.5–2 ng/mL for nocturnal erection [74]. Other studies describe other testosterone values: below 8.5 nmol/L for erectile dysfunction, below 11 nmol/L for decreased frequency of morning erections and below 13 nmol/L for diminished vigor [75].

Because of all this individual variability and also because of different testosterone thresholds for different symptoms, there is still no consensus from the major professional societies about the definition of hypogonadism [76–78].

3.1. Hypogonadism types

There are several types of hypogonadism that all lead to alteration of testosterone effects on target cells:

- Primary hypogonadism is due to different testicular causes: chromosomal diseases (Klinefelter syndrome being the most frequent disease [79]) or testicular tumors with testosterone deficiency after treatment [80]. Orchitis, acquired anorchia, indiopathic testicular atrophy, congenital anorchia, 46 XY sexual development disorders, gonadal dysgenetic syndrome,

Noonan Syndrome or LH receptor mutations are other causes of possible primary hypogonadism [76].

- Secondary hypogonadism is due to central, hypothalamic or hypophyseal causes: functional or tumoral hyperprolactinemia, Kallmann syndrome, isolated LH deficiency, pituitary adenomas, autoimmune hypophysitis, iatrogenic pituitary insufficient (surgery, radiotherapy), CNS tumors Prader-Willi syndrome, congenital adrenal hyperplasia [76].

Both gonad and hypothalamus insufficiency: late onset hypogonadism due to aging or overweight or both is a typical mechanism that is seen in late onset hypogonadism. The hypothalamic pulsatile secretion of gonadotropin-releasing hormone is blunted, due to increased hypothalamic sensitivity to negative feedback from the peripheral androgens, with preservation of the responsiveness of the pituitary gonadotrophs. From a peripheral point of view, testicular volume as well as Leydig cell mass and reserve function are diminished. There is a reduced testosterone secretion with associated loss of nycthemeral variability [81]. The combined defects are responsible for a progressive decrease of testosterone level with 1–2% per year [14]. Chronic ill men, obesity and metabolic syndrome also determine testosterone deficiency in high percentages with a variable prevalence of 25% [82] up to 50% [83]. Taken all into consideration up to 20% of all men over 60 years of age have inappropriate testosterone levels [84].

- Androgen receptor insensitivity/resistance is a very rare form of hypogonadism, due to total or partial androgen receptor insensitivity or 5-alpha reductase deficiency.

Regardless of type of hypogonadism, the clinical picture is dependent on the moment of onset of hypogonadism.

Prenatal testosterone deficiency will alter genital development, inducing all possible alteration of external genital aspects and formation: hypospadias, with different severity degrees, cryptorhidia, and ambiguous external genitals to female external genitals. These anatomical changes will impair future sexual function. The changes are irreversible and need surgical treatment for correction. The general surgical rule is to make the surgical treatment as soon as possible and to choose the gender, which is easier to be achieved with reconstructive treatment [85] but also in accordance to the intrauterine hormonal exposure. The goal is to complete the surgical correction till the age of 2 [86]. It is also important to evaluate, in the presence of nonfunctional/dysgenetic gonads, to evaluate the malignancy potential and to make the right treatment choices [87]. The major problems in many cases are unrecognized and undiagnosed at birth and are difficult to treat after 2 years of age because of organic causes and also due to the already established gender identity, gender role and sexual orientation. Testosterone replacement treatment is imperative, following the moment of physiological onset.

In cases of prepubertal testosterone deficiency, we will always observe a delayed puberty, defined in boys as no secondary sexual characters (increase in testes) before the age of 14 [88]. In severe causes of hypogonadism, the clinical picture is typical: small testes, cryptorhidia, gynecomastia, high-pitched voice, constant linear growth, eunuchoid habitus, sparse body and facial hair, decreased bone and muscle mass. From a sexuality point of view, these boys do not show sexual interest, have a decreased tendency of autostimulation, and have decreased phantasies and dreams. Untreated hypogonadism will affect all the levels of sexuality, with no normal development of sexuality. In the absence of normal androgen impregnation, there will be no erectile performance, altered sexual behavior, altered sense of well-being and globally affected sexual function [89]. If untreated, there will be no normal development of an adult male phenotype with serious impairment of sexual life.

Adult onset testosterone deficiency will induce different symptoms compared to previously mentioned forms of hypogonadism. The patients have normal developed genitals, normal developed secondary sexual characters, normal sexual function and behavior till the onset of hypogonadism. The clinical picture is dominated by metabolic and sexual symptoms. Sexual symptoms include loss of libido, erectile dysfunction, decrease in sexual phantasies, loss of body hair and hot flushes. Metabolic complications are loss of bone mass, sarcopenia, weight gain, increased body fat and increased vascular risk [90–92].

4. Treatment principles in testosterone deficiency in males

4.1. Life style changes

Life style changes are important only in late-onset hypogonadism, significant weight reduction, decrease of body fat and regular exercise can increase endogenous testosterone level [93, 94]. Life style changes can improve testosterone balance, in absence of active hormonal replacement treatment [95, 96] but unfortunately significant weight loss of more than 10% is difficult to maintain [96]. This is the motif for which, in majority of cases, supplemental treatment is needed [97]. Even if possible results are interesting, in the testosterone normalization in diabetic and overweight patients with metabolic syndrome (what is this?), the compliance to sustained weight reduction is low in the long run, so decreased testosterone will reappear whenever a new weight increase occurs. Testosterone deficiency prevention is still a goal, with management and treatment of modifiable factors, such as weight control, regular sport activities, and decreased alcohol consumption, but in the majority of cases, it is difficult to sustain.

4.2. Testosterone supplemental therapy

Currently, testosterone supplemental therapy is the golden standard for management of testosterone deficiency symptoms, regardless of physical, psychological or sexual domains [98].

There is no clear consensus for an accepted lower limit of normal testosterone. Various guidelines for the diagnosis of hypogonadism are available: late-onset hypogonadism [78] (total testosterone < 8 nmol/L) should be treated with testosterone therapy, those with total testosterone level of 8–12 nmol/L and hypogonadal symptoms should be given a trial of testosterone replacement therapy, and those with total testosterone level > 12 nmol/L are not hypogonadal and should not be treated [99]. Other guidelines recommend treatment for values below 8 nmol/L only in cases of physical symptoms [76, 100].

Testosterone measurements should be measured in the morning, between 07 and 11 AM, on two different days, and both values should be low in order to confirm the testosterone deficiency. Total testosterone measurements are used in order to make a positive diagnosis.

Interventional studies have shown a beneficial effect of testosterone replacement therapy on insulin resistance [101]. The increase in insulin sensitivity is present in obese men [102, 103], patients with heart failure [104], with better glycemic controls in diabetic males under testosterone replacement therapy [105, 106].

There are some recommendations of active testosterone screening in special risk categories of males [76, 100, 107]:

1. Type-2 diabetes mellitus
2. Metabolic syndrome
3. Moderate to severe chronic lung disease
4. Osteoporosis
5. History of infertility
6. Treatment with steroids, opiates and anticonvulsants
7. Alcohol abuse
8. ED or loss of spontaneous erections
9. Loss of sexual desire

The debate is around the type of symptoms that should be addressed for treatment. If correctly screened, with validated questionnaires, less than 5% of men with type-2 diabetes is asymptomatic, free of altered erectile performance, no present ED or altered arousal capacity [108].

The main concern in recommended testosterone replacement therapy is the vascular safety [109–111] because of the suggestion of increased stroke risk, despite the reduction in major adverse cardiovascular events, as death, nonfatal myocardial infarction and stroke. Some studies suggest beneficial effects of testosterone on cardiovascular risk factors [112], low testosterone being associated with increased cardiac mortality [113, 114].

The benefits for the cardio metabolic risk profile are clear, not only in the direction of insulin sensitivity, as seen before, but untreated testosterone deficiency is also associated with a fourfold risk of developing type-2 diabetes in men [97]. Some studies suggest that testosterone replacement therapy induces favorable changes in total and low-density lipoprotein profile, lipoprotein, body fat composition and glycated hemoglobin levels [108, 115, 116].

Recent studies showed different results suggesting an increase in vascular events in the presence of testosterone supplemental therapy [117–119]. Because of this opposing data, the FDA (Food and Drug Administration) still recommends that larger interventional studies are needed to have a definitive conclusion regarding testosterone treatment on cardiac safety [120]. Observational studies did not confirm the increase in cardiovascular events in long-term follow-up studies [121]. The EMA (European Medicines Agency) had agreed by consensus that there is no consistent evidence of an increased risk for heart problems with testosterone replacement in men lacking the hormone [122].

However, caution should be taken in cases with preexisting cardiovascular disease, especially in cases with increased hematocrit levels, due to increased primary thrombotic risk [123, 124].

Similar unresolved issues are seen when evaluating the associated presence of the following:

- Obstructive sleep apnea, classically considered a contraindication for testosterone treatment, because of neutral studies, with no worsening of the disease [125–127]
- Lower urinary tract symptoms, which do not worsen under testosterone treatment, as classically considered [128–130]
- Congestive heart failure is still a relative contraindications for replacement treatment, but controversial, since excellent results are seen in testosterone treatment in cases with well controlled congestive heart failure [131]. Maybe untreated/uncontrolled heart failure should be considered as a contraindication.
- Prostate safety: Prostate cancer is still a contraindication, but positive results start to emerge [76] with respect to lack of increased risk of prostate cancer under supplemental therapy. Also symptomatic hypogonadal men with localized prostate cancer, treated surgically, without active disease can be cautiously considered for testosterone therapy [132–134]

Taking all these recommendations into consideration, testosterone has clear benefits regarding sexual health [97]. There is a significant effect on sexual desire, intercourse satisfaction and overall sexual satisfaction, when evaluated with FSFI questionnaire [135]. There are clear benefits on erectile function, with satisfactory sexual intercourses after at least 3 months of testosterone supplementation [135, 136]. Also, testosterone treatment, in hypogonadal men, improves the therapeutical response to phosphodiesterase-5 inhibitors [137], converting non-responders to responders [138]. In general, testosterone supplementation has a positive effect on orgasmic and ejaculatory function [139]. Sexual interest appears after the first 3 weeks of use and reaches plateau in 6 weeks [136].

Except the late-onset hypogonadism, classical indications for testosterone supplementation are delayed puberty, Klinefelter syndrome, low bone mass in adult hypogonadism, hypopituitarism, and testicular dysgenesis. The therapy should be started at the appropriate age of puberty onset (in prepubertal forms of diseases) or after the clear diagnosis of hypogonadism (in postpubertal forms of diseases) [76]. Active follow-up should be performed in patients treated with testosterone supplementation therapy [76, 140]:

- Symptoms response at every visit, minimum after 3 months of treatment, and then annually.
- Formulation of specific adverse effects should be evaluated at each visit.
- Testosterone level should be measured periodically, for a correct supplemental therapy at 3, 6 and 12 months after onset of the treatment.
- All and each adverse event should be reported immediately.
- Bone mineral density should be measured every 1–2 years
- PSA measurement should be performed every 3 months, in the 1st year of treatment and then annually

- Hematocrit measurement should be monitored at 3, 6 and 12 months and, thereafter, annually. Whenever the levels increase above 0.54, testosterone treatment should be discontinued.

5. Conclusion

When we think about hypogonadism, we should keep in mind not only the classical types of hypogonadism due to classical testicular disease of central, hypothalamic and hypophyseal disease, but we should also emphasize the partial testosterone deficiency that is described due to age increase (late-onset hypogonadism) or secondary to weight increase (up to 30% of males with metabolic syndrome and 50% of males with diabetes) or the secondary hypogonadism described after chronic use of steroids or after long exposure to stress, especially in young males. All these types of hypogonadism that affect young, middle-aged or old males are presented separately. The therapeutic approach should be individualized for each type of hypogonadism and should consider positive and possible negative effects. All alternatives are presented: life style changes, sustained weight loss, increased exercise, supplemental therapy and pro-fertility treatment.

Author details

Dana Stoian*, Ioana Mozos, Marius Craina, Corina Paul, Iulian Velea, Adalbert Schiller and Mihaela Craciunescu

*Address all correspondence to: stoian.dana@umft.ro

University of Medicine and Pharmacy: Victor Babes, Timisoara, Romania

References

[1] Smith CA, Sinclair AH. The cell biology and molecular genetics of testis determination. Results and Problem in Cell Differentiation. 2000;**28**:23-52

[2] Capel B. The battle of the sexes. Mechanisms of Development. 2000;**92**:89-10

[3] Josso N, Cate RL, Picard JY, Vigier B, di Clemente N, Wilson C, Imbeaud S, Pepinsky RB, Guerrier D, Boussin L. Anti-Müllerian hormone: The jost factor. Recent Progress in Hormone Research. 1993;**18**:1-59

[4] Siiteri PK, MacDonald PC. Role of extraglandular estrogen in human endocrinology. In: Greep RO, Astwood EB, editors. Handbook of Physiology, Vol. II. Female Reproductive System, Part I. Washington, DC: American Physiological Society; 1973. pp. 615-629

[5] Grumbach MM, Conte FA. Disorders of sex differentiation. In: Wilson JD, Foster DW, Kronenberg HM, Larsen PR, editors. Williams Textbook of Endocrinology. 9th ed. Philadelphia: W.B. Saunders Co; 1998. pp. 1303-1425

[6] Celec P, OStatnikova D, Hodosy J. On the effects of testosterone on brain behavioural functions. Frontiers in Neuroscience.2015;**912**. DOI: 10.3389/fnins.2015.00012

[7] Hiort O, Thyen U, Holterhus PM. The basis of gender assignment in disorders of somatosexual differentiation. Hormone Research. 2005;**64**:18-22

[8] Sex begins in the womb. Exporing the biological contributions to human health. Wizemann T, Pardue ML eds. Institute of Medicine (US) Comitee on Understanding the biology of sex and gender differences. Wizemann TM, Pardue ML, editors. Washingtopn (DC): National Academic Press (US): 2001

[9] Molina P. Male reproductive system. In: Molina P, editor. Endocrine Physiology. 4th ed. Mc Graw Hill Co; 2013. USA

[10] Feldman HA, Goldstein I, HAtzichristou, et al. Impotence and its medical and psychosocial correlates: Results of the Massachuses Male Aging Study. Journal of Urology. 1994;**151**:54-61

[11] Braun M, Wassmer G, Klotz T, Reifenrath B, Mathers M, Engelmann U. Epidemiology of erectile dysfunction: Results of the Cologne Male Survey. International Journal of Impotence Research. 2000;**12**:305

[12] Vermeulen A. Andropause. Maturitas. 2000;**34**:5-15

[13] Harman SM, Metter EJ, Tobin JD, Pearson J, Blackman MR. Baltimore Longitudinal Study of Aging. Longitudinal effects of aging on serum total and free testosterone levels in healthy men. Baltimore Longitudinal Study of Aging. Journal of Clinical Endocrinology and Metabolism. 2001;**86**(2):724-731

[14] Feldman HA, Longcope C, Derby CA, Johannes CB, Araujo AB, Coviello AD, Bremner WJ, McKinlay JB. Age trends in the level of serum testosterone and other hormones in middle-aged men: Longitudinal results from the Massachusetts male aging study. Journal of Clinical Endocrinology and Metabolism. 2002;**87**(2):589-598

[15] Stanworth RD, Hugh Jones T. Testosterone for the aging male; current evidence and recommended practice. Clinical Interventions in Aging. 2008;**3**(1):25-44

[16] Tran TS, Center JR, Seibel MJ, Eisman JA, Kushnir MM, Rockwood AL, Nyuyen TV. Relationship between serum testosterone and Fracture risk in men: A comparison of RIA and LC0 MS/MS. Clinical Chemistry. 2015;**61**(9):1182-1190

[17] Traish AM. Testosterone therapy in men with testostosterone deficiency: Are we beyond the point of no return? Investigative and Clinical Urology. 2016;**57**(6):384-400

[18] Ogawa S. Role of androgen in the elderly. Frailty and androgens. Clinical Calcium. 2013;**23**(8):1117-1122

[19] Svartberg J, von Muhlen D, Schirmer H, Barrett-Connor E, Sundfjord J, Jorde R. Association of endogenous testosterone with blood pressure and left ventricular mass in men. The Tromsø Study. European Journal of Endocrinology. 2004;**150**(1):65-71

[20] Naifar M, Rekik N, Messedi M, Chaabouni K, Lahiani A, Turk M, Abid M, Ayedi F, Jamoussi K. Male hypogonadism and metabolic syndrome. Andrologia. 2015;**47**(5):579-586

[21] Santos MR, Sayegh AL, Groehs RV, Fonseca G, Trombetta IC, BAretto AC, Arap MA, Negrao CE, Middlekauff HR, Alves MJ. ARQUIVOS Brasileiros De Cardiologia. 2015;**105**(3):256-264

[22] Pye SR, Huhtaniemi IT, Finn JD, Lee DM, O'Neil TW, Tajar A, BArtfai G, Boonen S, CAsanueva FF, Forti G, Giwercman A, Han TS, Kula K, Lean ME, Pendleton N, Punab M, Rutter MK, Vanderschueren D, Wu FC; EMAS Study Group. Late onset hypogonadism and mortality in aging male. Journal of Clinical Endocrinology & Metabolism. 2014;**99**(4):1357-1366

[23] Muralledharan V, Marsh H, Kapoor D, Channer KS, Jones TH. Testosterone deficiency is associated with increased risk of mortality and testosterone replacement improves survival in men with type 2 diabetes. European Journal of Endocrinology. 2013;**169**(6):725-733

[24] Masters W, Johnson V, Kolodny R, editors. Childhood Sexuality in in Human Sexuality. 5th ed. New York: Logman Inc.; 1995

[25] Carthy MM, et al. Sexual differentiation of the brain: Mode, mechanisms, and meaning. In: Pfaff DW, et al., editors. Hormones, Brain and Behaviour. 2nd ed. Academic Press; US; 2009. pp. 1707-1744

[26] Hines M. Sex-related variation in human behaviour and the brain. Trends in Cognitive Sciences. 2010;**14**(10):448-456

[27] Reinisch JM. Prenatal exposure to synthetic progestin increases potential for aggression in humans. Science. 1981;**211**(4487):1171-1173

[28] Ehrhardt AA, Money J. Progestin-induced hermaphroditism: IQ and psychosexual identity in a study of ten girls. The Journal of Sex Research. 1967;**3**:83-100

[29] Ehrhardt AA, et al. Prenatal exposure to medroxyprogesterone acetate (MPA) in girls. Psychoneuroendocrinology. 1977;**2**:391-398

[30] Hines M, et al. Testosterone during pregnancy and childhood gender role behavior: A longitudinal population study. Child Development. 2002;**73**:1678-1687

[31] Alexander GM, Hines M. Sex differences in response to children's toys in nonhuman primates (cercopithecus aethiops sabaeus). Evolution and Human Behaviour. 2002;**23**:467-479

[32] Alexander GM. An evolutionary perspective of sex-typed toy preferences: Pink, blue, and the brain. Archives of Sexual Behaviour. 2003;**32**:7-14

[33] Hines M. Brain Gender. Oxford University Press, UK; 2004

[34] Hines M, et al. Androgen and psychosexual development: Core gender identity, sexual orientation and recalled childhood gender role behaviour in women and men with congenital adrenal hyperplasia (CAH). Journal of Sex Research. 2004;**41**:1-7

[35] Ehrhardt AA, Baker SW. Fetal androgens, human central nervous system differentiation, and behaviour sex differences. In: New York. pp. 33-52

[36] Brooks-Gunn J, Graber JA, Paikoff RL. Studying links between hormones and negative affect: Models and measures. Journal of Research on Adolescence. 1994;**4**:469-486

[37] Buchanan CM, Eccles JS, Becker JB. Are adolescents the victims of raging hormones: Evidence for activational effects of hormones on moods and behaviour at adolescence. Psychological Bulletin. 1992;**111**:62-10

[38] Spear LP. Neurobehavioral changes in adolescence. Current Directions in Psychologi cal Science. 2000;**9**:111-114

[39] Crouter AC, Manke BA, McHale SM. The family context of gender intensification in early adolescence. Child Development. 1995; **66**:317-329

[40] Hill JP, Lynch ME. The intensification of gender-related role expectations during early adolescence. In: Brooks-Gunn J, Petersen AC, editors. Girls at Puberty: Biological and Psychosocial Perspectives. New York: Plenum Press; 1983. pp. 201-228

[41] Kent A. Testosterone and sexual drive. Reviews in Obstetrics and Gynecology 2009; **2**(1):65-66

[42] Masters WE, Johnson VE, Kolodny RC. Sexual physiology, in Human Sexuality, Masters 5th Ed. J, Johnson V, Kolodny R eds. 1995. New York: Longman Inc., US

[43] Goldey KL, Avery LR, van Anders S. Sexual fantasies and gender/sex: A multi method approach with quantitative content analysis and hormonal response. Journal of Sex Research. 2014;**5**(8):917-931

[44] Brett M.A., Roberts L.F., Johnson T.W. Eunuchs in contemporary society: Expectations, consequences, and adjustments to castration (part II) J Sex Med. 2007;**4**:946

[45] Wibowo E, Wassersug R, Warkentin K. Impact of androgen deprivation therapy on sexual function: A response. Asian Journal of Andrology. 2012;**14**:793

[46] Handy AB, Jackowich RA, Wibovo E, Johnson TW, Wassersug RJ. FGender preference in the sexual attraction, Fantasies and relationship of voluntarily castrated men. Sex Med 2016 **4** (1): e51-59

[47] Corona G, RAstrelli G, Ricca V, Jannini EA, Vignozzi L, Monani M, Sforza A, Forti G, Mannucci E, Maggi M. Risk factors associated with primary and secondary reduced libido in male patients with sexual dysfunction. Journal of Sexual Medicine. 2013; **10**(4):1074-1089

[48] Lejeune H, Huyghe E, Droupy S. Hypoactive sexual desire and testosterone deficiency in men. Progress of Urology. 2013;**23**(9):621-628

[49] Corona G, Rastrelli G, Vignozzi L, Mannucci E, Maggi M. How to recognize late onset hypogonadism in men wuth sexual dysfunction. Asian Journal of Andrology. 2012;**14**(2):251-259

[50] Dean RC, Lue TF. Physiology of penile erection and pathophysiology of erectile dysfunction. Urologic Clinics of North America. 2005;**32**(4):379

[51] Stoleru S, Redoute J, Costes N, et al. Brain processing of visual sexual stimuli in men with hypoactive sexual desire disorder. Psychiatry Research. 2003;**124**:67

[52] Mouras H, Stoleru S, Bittoun J, et al. Brain processing of visual sexual stimuli in healthy men: A functional magnetic resonance imaging study. Neuroimage. 2003;**20**:855

[53] Arnow BA, Desmond JE, Banner LL, et al. Brain activation and sexual arousal in healthy, heterosexual males. Brain. 2002;**125**:1014

[54] Burnett AL. Neurophysiology of erectile function: Androgenic effects. Journal of Andrology. 2003;**24**:S2-S5

[55] Saenz de Tejada I. Further commentary: Physiology of erectile function and pathophysiology of erectile dysfunction. In: Lue TF, Basson R, Rosen R, Giuliano F, Khoury S, Montorsi F, editors. The Second International Consultation on Sexual Medicine: Sexual Medicine-Sexual dysfunctions in Men and Women. Plymouth: Plymbridge Distributors Ltd.; 2004. pp. 289-343

[56] Purves Tyson TD, Handelsman DJ, Double KL, Owens SJ, Bustamante S, Weickert CS. Testosterone regulation of sex steroid related mRNAs and dopamine-related mRNAs in adolescent male rat substantia nigra. BMC Neuroscience. 2012;**13**:95. DOI: 10.1186/1471-2202-12-95

[57] Meisel RL, Sachs BD. The physiology of male sexual behaviour. In: Knobil E, Neill JGS, Greenwald GS, Markert CL, Pfaff DW, editors. The Physiology of Reproduction. Vol. 2. New York: Raven Press; 1994. pp. 3-107

[58] Mills TM, Reilly CM, Lewis RW. Androgens and penile erection: A review. Journal of Andrology. 1996;**17**:633-638

[59] Baba K, Yajima M, Carrier S. Effect of testosterone on nitric oxide synthetase-containing nerve fibres and intracavernous pressure in rat corpus cavernosum. International Journal of Impotence Research. 1994;**6**:S1. D6

[60] Takahashi Y, Hirata Y, Yokoyama S, Ishii N, Nunes L, Lue TF, Tanagho EA. Loss of penile erectile response to intracavernous injection of acetylcholine in castrated dog. The Tohoku Journal of Experimental Medicine. 1991;**163**:85-91

[61] Zvara P, Sioufi R, Schipper HM, Begin LR, Brock GB. Nitric oxide mediated erectile activity is a testosterone dependent event: A rat erection model. International Journal of Impotence Research. 1995;**7**:209-219

[62] Shabsigh R. The effect of testosterone on the cavernous tissue and erectile function. World Journal of Urology. 1997;**15**(1):21-26

[63] Mann K, Sohn M. Spontaneous noctrumnal erection physiologic and clinical applications. Somnologie. 2005;**9**(3):119-126

[64] Carani C, Bancroft J, Granata A, Del Rio G, Marrama P. testosterone and erectile function, nocturnal penile tumescence and rigidity, and erectile response to visual erotic stimuli in hypogonadal and Eugonadal men. Psychoneuroendrocrinology. 1992;**17**(6):647-654

[65] Husnu T, Ersoz A, Bulent E, Tacettin O, Remzi A, Bulent A, Aydin M. Obstructive sleep apnea syndrome and erectile dysfunction: Does long term continuous positive pressure improve erections. African Health Sciences. 2015;**15**(1):171-179

[66] Levine SB. The nature of sexual desire: A clinician's perspective. Archives of Sexual Behavior. 2003;**32**(3):279-285

[67] Morales A, Buvat J, Gooren LJ, Guay AT, Kaufmann JM, Kim YC, Tan HM, Torres LO. Endocrine aspects of men sexual dysfunction. In: Lue TF, Basson R, Rosen R, Guiliano F, Khoury S, Montorsi F, editors. Sexual Medicine: Sexual Dysfunction in Men and Women 2nd International Consultation on Sexual Dysfunction. Paris: Health Publication; 2004

[68] Barkin J. Erectile dysfunction and hypogonadism. Canadian Journal of Urology. 2011; **18**(S2):7

[69] Buvat J, Bou Jaoude G. Significance of hypogonadism in erectile dysfunction. World Journal of Urology. 2006;**24**(6):657-667

[70] Morales A, Biuvat J, Gooren LJ, Guat AT, Kaufman JM, Tan HM, Torres LO. Endocrine aspects of sexual dysfunction in men. The Journal of Sexual Medicine. 2004;**1**(1):69-81

[71] Zitzmann M, Faber S, Nieschlag E. Association of specific symptoms and metabolic risk with serum testosterone in older men. Journal of Clinical Endocrinology & Metabolism. 2006;**91**(11):4335-4343

[72] Gray PB, Singh AB, Woodhouse LJ, et al. Dose-dependent effects of testosterone on sexual function, mood, and visuospatial cognition in older men. Journal of Clinical Endocrinology & Metabolism. 2005;**90**:3838-3846

[73] Kelleher S, Conway AJ, Handelsman DJ. Blood testosterone thersold for androgen deficiency symptoms. Journal of Clinical Endocrinology & Metabolism. 2004;**69**(8):3813-3817

[74] Carani C, Zini D, Baldini A, et al. Testosterone and prolactin: behavioural and psychophysiological approaches in men. In: Bancroft J, et al., editors. The Pharmacology of Sexual Function and Dysfunction. Amsterdam: Elsevier Science; 1995. pp. 145-150

[75] Vesper HW. Interlaboratory comparison study of serum total testosterone measurements performed by mass spectrometry methods. Steroids. 2009;**74**(6):498-503

[76] Dohle GR, Arver S, Bettocchi C, Joones TH, Kliesch S, Punab M. Guidelines on Male Hypogonadism. EAU. 2015. Available from: http://www.uroweb.org/guidelines/online-guidelines/

[77] Petak SV, Nankin HR, Spark RF, swerdloff RS, Rodriquez Rihgau. AACE Guidelines for evaluation and treatment of hypogonadism in adult male patients. Endocrine Practice. 2002;**8**(6):439-456

[78] Bhasin S, Cunningham GR, Hayes FJ, Matsumoto AM, Snyder PJ, Swerdloff RS, Montori VM. Testosterone therapy in men with androgen deficiency syndromes: an endocrine clinical practice guide. 2010;**95**(6): 2536-2559

[79] Bojesen A, et al. Prenatal and postnatal prevalence of Klinefelter syndrome: A national registry study. Journal of Clinical Endocrinology & Metabolism. 2003;**88**(2):622-626

[80] Eberhart J, et al. Risk factors for postreatment hypogonadism in testicular cancer patients. European Journal of Endocrinology. 2008;**158**(4):561-570

[81] Mahmoud A, Comhaire FH. Mechanisms of disease: Late-onset hypogonadism. Nature Clinical Practice Urology. 2006;**3**(8):430-438

[82] Dandona P, Dhindsa S. hypogonadotropic hypogonadism in type 2 diabetes and obesity. JCEM. 2011; **96**(9):2643-2651

[83] Kapoor D, Aldred H, Clark S, Channer KS, Jones H. Clinical and biochemical assessment of hypogonadism in men with type 2 diabetes. Diabetes Care. 2007;**30**(4):911-917

[84] Kaufmann J, Vermeulen A. The decline of androgens levels in elderly men and its clinical implications. Endocrine Reviews. 2005;**26**:833-876

[85] Moshiri M, Chapman MD, Fechner PY, Dubinsky TJ, Shnohavorian M, Osman S, Bharga P, Katz DS. Evaluation an management of disorders of sexual development: multidisciplinary approach to a complex diagnosis. Radiographics 2012;**32**(6):1599-1618

[86] Göllü G, Yildiz RV, Bingol-Kologlu M, et al. Ambiguous genitalia: An overview of 17 years' experience. Journal of Pediatric Surgery. 2007;**42**(5):840-844

[87] Looijenga LHJ, Hersmus R, Oosterhuis JW, Cools M, Drop SL, Wolffenbuttel KP. Tumor risk in disorders of sex development (DSD). Best Practice & Research: Clinical Endocrinology & Metabolism. 2007;**21**(3):480-495

[88] Palmert MR, Dunkel L. Delaued puberty. The New England Journal of Medicine. 2012; **366**:4430453

[89] Kumar P, Kumar N, Thakur DS, Patidar A. Male Hypogonadism symptoms and treatment. Journal of Advanced Pharmaceutical Technology & Research. 2010;**1**(3):297-301

[90] Laughin A, Barret-Connor E, Bergstrom J. Low serum testosterone and mortality in older men. Journal of Clinical Endocrinology & Metabolism. 2008;**93**:68-75

[91] Travosin TG, Shackelton R, Arujo AB. The natural history of symptomatic androgen deficiency in men: Onset, progression, and spontaneous remission. Journal of the American Geriatrics Society. 2008;**56**:831-839

[92] Arujo AB, Esche GR, Kepulian V, et al. Prevalence of symptomatic androgen deficiency in men. Journal of Clinical Endocrinology & Metabolism. 2007;**92**:4241-4247

[93] Kumagai H, Zempo-Miyaki A, Yoshikawa T, Tsujimoto T, Tanaka K, Maeda S. Lifestyle modification increases serum testosterone level and decrease central blood pressure in overweight and obese men. Endocrine Journal. 2015;**62**(95):423-430

[94] Bobadilla L, Aberg K, Johnson M, Shirtcliff EA. Experiences in the military may impact dual axis neuroendocrine processes in veterans. Developmental Psychobiology. 2015;**57**(6):719-730

[95] Moro T, Tinsley G, Bianco A, Marcolin G, Pacelli QF, Battaglia G, Palma A, Gentil P, Neri M, Paoli A. Effects of eight weeks of time-restricted feeding (16/8) on basal metabolism, maximal strength, body composition, inflammation, and cardiovascular risk factors in resistance-trained males. Journal of Translational Medicine. 2016;**14**(1):290

[96] Cunnigham GR. Testosterone and metabolic syndrome. Asian Journal of Andrology. 2015;**17**(2):192-196

[97] Hackett G. An update on the role of testosterone replacement therapy in the management of hypogonadism. Therapeutic Advances in Irology. 2016;**8**(2):147-160

[98] Hissaues S. Contemporary perspective and management of testosterone deficiency: Modifiable factors and variable management. International Journal of Urology. 2015; **22**(12):1084-1095

[99] Nieschlag E, Swerdloff R, Behre HM, Gooren LJ, Kaufman JM, Legros JJ, Lunenfeld B, Morley JE, Schulman C, Wang C, Weidner W, Wu FC: Investigation, treatment and monitoring of late-onset hypogonadism in males: ISA, ISSAM, and EAU recommendations. International Journal of Andrology. 2005;**28**:125-127

[100] Wylie R, Rees M, Hacket G, Anderson R, Bouloux P, Cust M. Androgens, health and sexuality in women and men. Maturitars. 2010;**67**:275-289

[101] Simon D, Charles MA, Lahlou N, Nahoul K, Oppert JM, Gouault-Heilmann M, Lemort N, Thibult N, Joubert E, Balkau B, Eschwege E. Androgen therapy improves insulin sensitivity and decreases leptin level in healthy adult men with low plasma total testosterone. Diabetes Care. 2001;**24**:2149-2151

[102] Marin P, Holmang S, Jonsson L, Sjostrom L, Kvist H, Holm G, Lindstedt G, Bjorntorp P. The effects of testosterone treatment on body composition and metabolism in middle-aged obese men. International Journal of Obesity and Related Metabolic Disorders. 1992;**16**:991-997

[103] Marin P, Krotkiewski M, Bjorntorp P. Androgen treatment of middle-aged, obese men: Effects on metabolism, muscle and adipose tissues. European Journal of Medicinal. 1992;**1**:329-336

[104] Malkin CJ, Jones TH, Channer KS. The effect of testosterone on insulin sensitivity in men with heart failure. European Journal of Heart Failure. 2007;**9**:40-50

[105] Kapoor D, Goodwin E, Channer KS, Jones TH. Testosterone replacement therapy improves insulin resistance, glycaemic control, visceral adiposity and hypercholesterolemia in hypogonadal men with type 2 diabetes. European Journal of Endocrinology. 2006;**154**:899-906

[106] Boyanov MA, Boneva Z, Christov VG. Testosterone supplementation in men with type 2 diabetes, visceral obesity and partial androgen deficiency. Aging Male. 2003;**6**:1-7

[107] Home P, MAnt J, Diaz J, Turner C Guideline development group. Management of type 2 diabetes summary of update NICE guidance. British Medical Journal. 2008; **336**:1306-1308

[108] Hacket G, Cole N, Bhartia M, Wilkinson P, Raju J, Wilkinson P. Testosterone replacement therapy improves metabolic parameters in hypogonadal men with type 2 diabetes but not in men with coexisting depression the BLAST study. Journal of Sexual Medicine. 2014;**11**:840-856

[109] Anderson JL, May HT, Lappe DL, Bair T, Le V, Carquist JF, Muhlestein JB. Impact of testosterone replacement therapy in myocardial infarction, stroke and death in men with low testosterone concentrations in an integrated health care system. American Journal of Cardiology. 2016;**117**(5):794-799

[110] Kloner RA, Carson C, Dobs A, Kopecky S, Mohler ER. Testosterone and cardiovascular disease. Journal of the American College of Cardiology. 2016;**67**(5):5450557

[111] Traish AM, Zitzmann M. The complex and multifactorial relationship between testosterone deficiency obesity and vascular disease. Reviews in Endocrine and Metabolic Disorders. 2015;**16**(3):249-268

[112] Jones TH. Testosterone deficiency: A risk factor for cardiovascular disease? Trends in Endocrinology and Metabolism. 2010;**21**(8):496-503

[113] Corona G. Hypogonadism as a risk factor for cardiovascular mortality in men. Meta analytic study. European Journal of Endocrinology. 2011;**165**(5):687-701

[114] Malkin CJ. Low serum testosterone and increased mortality in men with coronary heart disease. Heart. 2010;**96**(22):1821-1825

[115] Traish A, Haider A, Doros G, Saad F. Long term testosterone therapy in hypogonadal men ameliorates elements of metabolic syndrome: An observational, long term registry study. International Journal of Clinical Practice. 2014;**68**:314-329

[116] Saad F, Yassin A, Haider A, Doros G, Gooren L. Elderly men over 65 years o age with late onset hypogonadism benefits as much from testosterone treatment as do younger men. Jorrean Journal of Urology. 2015;**56**:310-317

[117] Basaria S. Adverse events associated with testosterone administration. The New England Journal of Medicine. 2010;**363**(2):109-122

[118] Finkle WD. Increase risk of nonfatal myocardial infarction following testosterone therapy prescription in men. PLoS One. 2014;**9**(1):e85805

[119] Vigen R. Association of testosterone therapy with mortality, myocardial infarction, and stroke in men with low testosterone levels. Journal of the American Medical Association. 2013;**310**(17):1829-1836

[120] FDA. Advisory committee industry briefing document. Testosterone therapy. Bone, reproductive and urologic drug advisory committee and the drug safety and risk management advisory committee. 2014

[121] Baillargeon J. Risk of myocardial infarction in older men receiving testosterone therapy. Annals of Pharmacotherapy. 2014;**48**(9):1138-1144

[122] Review of testosterone containing medicine started. EMA/209962/2014. European Medicine Agency 2014. Available from: www.ema.europa.eu/docs

[123] Gagnon DR. Hematocrit and risk of cardiovascular disease – the Framingham study: A 34-year follow up. American Heart Journal. 1994;**127**(3):674-682

[124] Boffetta PA. U shaped relationship between haematocrit and mortality in a large prospective cohort study. International Journal of Epidemiology. 2013;**42**(2):601-615

[125] Hildreth KL, Barry DW, Moreau KL, et al. Effects of testosterone and progressive resistance exercise in healthy, highly functioning older men with low normal testosterone levels. Journal of Clinical Endocrinology & Metabolism. 2013;**98**(5):1891-1990

[126] Hoyos CM, Killock R, Yee BJ. Effects of testosterone therapy on sleep and breathing in obese men with severe obstructive sleep apnoea: A randomized controlled trial. Clinical Endocrinology (Oxford). 2012;**77**(4):599-607

[127] Killick R, Wang D, Hoyos CM. The effects of testosterone on ventilatory responses in men with obstructive slpee apnea: A randomised, placebo controlled trial. Journal of Sleep Research. 2013;**22**(3):331-336

[128] Kalichenko SY, Tishova YA, Maskhlaya GJ. Effects of testosterone supplementation on markers of the metabolic syndrome and inflammation in hypogonadal men with metabolic syndrome: The double blind placebo controlled Moscow study. Clinical Endocrinology (Oxford). 2010;**73**(5):602-612

[129] Srinivas Shankar U, Roberts SA, Connolly MJ. Effects of testosterone on muscle strength, physical activity, body composition, and quality of life in intermediate frail and frail elderly men: A randomized, double blind, placebo controlled study. Journal of Clinical Endocrinology & Metabolism. 2010;**95**(5):639-650

[130] Tan WS, Low WY, Ng CJ. Efficacy and safety on long acting intramuscular testosterone undecanoate in aging men: A randomised controlled study. BJU International. 2013;**111**(7):1130-1140

[131] Stout M, tew GA, Doll H. Testosterone therapy during exercise rehabilitation in males with chronic heart failure who have low testosterone status: A double blind randomized controlled feasibility study. American Heart Journal. 2012;**164**(6):893-901

[132] Morgentaler A. Testosterone therapy in men with prostate cancer: Scientific and ethical considerations. Journal of Urology. 2009;**181**(3):972-979

[133] Aversa A. Cardiometabolic complications after androgen deprivation therapy in men with prostate cancer: Effects of a 3 years intermittent testosterone supplementation. Frontiers in Endocrinology (Laussanne). 2012;**3**:17

[134] Kaufman JM. Androgen replacement after curative radical prostatectomy for prostate cancer in hypogonadal men. Journal of Urology. 2004;**172**(3):920-922

[135] Moon du G. The efficacy and safety of testosterone undecanoate in testosterone deficiency in Korea: A multicentre prospective study. Journal of Sexual Medicine. 2010;7(6):2253-2260

[136] Saad F. Onset of effects of testosterone treatment and time span until maximum effects are achieved. European Journal of Endocrinology. 2011;**165**(5):675-685

[137] Corona G. Testosterone supplementation and sexual function. A meta analysis study. Journal of Sexual Medicine. 2014;**11**(6):1577-1592

[138] Buvat J, Montorsi F, Maggi M, Porsst H, Kaipia A., Colson M. Hypogonadal men nonresponders to the PDE5 inhibitor Tadalafil benefit from normalization of testosterone gelin the treatment of erectile dysfunction. Journal of Sexual Medicine. 2011;**8**:284-293

[139] Boloña ER, Uraga MV, Haddad RM, Tracz MJ, Sideras K, Kennedy CC, Caples SM, Erwin PJ, Montori VM. Testosterone use in men with sexual dysfunction: A systematic review and meta-analysis of randomized placebo-controlled trials. Mayo Clinic Proceedings. 2007;**82**:20-28

[140] Dandona P, Rosenberg MT. A practical guide to male hypogonadism in the primary care setting. The International Journal of Clinical Practice. 2010;**64**(6):682-696

Section 4

Antidepressants and Sexual Dysfunction

Chapter 4

Sexual Dysfunction, Depression and Antidepressants: A Translational Approach

Jocelien D.A. Olivier, Diana C. Esquivel Franco,
Marcel D. Waldinger and Berend Olivier

Additional information is available at the end of the chapter

http://dx.doi.org/10.5772/intechopen.69105

Abstract

Major depression is frequently associated with sexual dysfunctions. Most antidepressants, especially selective serotonin reuptake inhibitors (SSRIs), induce additional sexual side effects and, although effective antidepressants, deteriorate sexual symptoms, which are the main reason that patients stop antidepressant treatment. Many strategies have been used to circumvent the additional sexual side effects, but results are rather disappointing. Recently, new antidepressants have been introduced, vilazodone and vortioxetine, which seem to lack sexual side effects in the early registration trials. Much research with large numbers of depressed patients and adequate methodological tools still has to confirm in daily use the absence of sexual side effects of new antidepressants. Animal models that in an early phase of drug development may predict putative sexual side effects of new antidepressants are extremely useful and could speed up development of new antidepressants. A rat model of sexual behavior is described that has a very high predictive validity for sexual side effects in man. Several characteristics of present antidepressants with regard to sexual dysfunctions are also present in the rat model and establish its validity. The animal model can also be used in the search for new psychotropics without sexual side effects or for drugs with sexual stimulating activity.

Keywords: depression, sexual dysfunction, antidepressants, sexual side effects, SSRI, animal model

1. Introduction: depression and sexual (dys)function

Sexual functioning in humans is a very complex phenomenon and involves many interacting processes that have been conceptualized as desire, arousal, and orgasm [1]. It is plausible to imagine that disturbances in the networks steering the appropriate processes may lead to disturbances in various aspects of sexual behavior or even to sexual dysfunction.

Major depression is often associated with sexual dysfunctions [2, 3]. Treatment of the depression with antidepressants complicates the situation considerably. Whereas some aspects of sexual functioning may improve, especially libido, others, notably erection and ejaculation may deteriorate. It is often difficult or impossible to ascertain what is caused by depression and what caused by the antidepressant, their interaction or even other factors. Lahon et al. [4] suggest that a complaint by a patient of sexual dysfunction might either indicate a failure to respond to treatment or the side effects of the drug. The large majority of commonly prescribed antidepressants are associated with sexual side effects, which often lead to noncompliance to the treatment. In an early study, Monteiro et al. [5] described that approx. 20% of patients treated with the tricyclic antidepressant clomipramine did stop treatment due to anorgasmia or delayed ejaculation. Although some clinicians were aware that antidepressants like tricyclics and monoamine oxidase (MAO) inhibitors induce sexual side effects [6], most clinicians were clearly unaware of such side effects. In the first decades of antidepressant use, other side effects like sedation, dizziness, hypotension, nausea, and anticholinergic effects were prominent. Only with the introduction of the serotonin reuptake inhibitors (SSRIs), these "old" side effects were no longer troublesome leading to an "explosive" use of this new, safe antidepressant class. Gradually, it became clear that SSRI use was associated with sexual side effects [7]. In the last decade, attempts were made to develop and introduce new antidepressants with low(er) sexual side effects, e.g., vilazodone and vortioxetine.

Clinically, drug-induced sexual dysfunction should be recognized because of noncompliance to the treatment [8], but on the other side, it also may complicate recovery from depression, e.g., by decreasing patient's self-esteem, self-worth, and competence and may put additional stress on relationships [9]. The latter authors give an excellent and extensive review on antidepressant-induced sexual dysfunction in men. This is an extremely complicated area because of the methodology used, the changes in the methodology over time, and the pharmacological differences in the various antidepressants and doses used. One of the most clear-cut differences, in the incidence of sexual side effects reported, has to do with instruments used to inquire about them. Montejo-González et al. [10] showed a fourfold difference in the percentage of patients reporting sexual dysfunction spontaneously versus reporting after direct inquiry by the clinician. Almost all double-blind, placebo-controlled drug trials of antidepressants are performed by pharmaceutical companies. They often compare their product with a competitive drug already present in the market. If sexual side effect incidence is an important factor in the future marketing of the drug, the pharmaceutical company often uses a competing antidepressant with a known, high propensity to induce sexual side effects. Although this may lead to the suggestion of a lower propensity to induce such effects, in later clinical practice realistic data are materialized and often lead to a different profile. Many more serious issues cloud the interpretations of many studies into the sexual side effects of antidepressants [9].

2. What are the sexual side effects of antidepressants in men?

Early antidepressants (tricyclic (TCA), heterocyclic, and (irreversible) monoamine oxidase inhibitors (MAOI)) have not very well been investigated regarding associated sexual side effects. Many case reports and small clinical studies have been performed, and the data suggested various sexual side effects [8]. Only two placebo-controlled studies were performed. Imipramine (a TCA) induced delayed orgasms in approx. 20–30% of the patients and phenelzine (an irreversible MAOI) in approx. 30–37% [11]. Monteiro et al. [5] found that after taking clomipramine, more than 90% of patients had difficulty in achieving orgasm. This study was performed in obsessive-compulsive disorder patients, a disorder not associated with basic sexual dysfunction itself. Although all these "classic" antidepressants have a polypharmacological mode of action, the high incidence of sexual side effects after clomipramine, the most "serotonergic" TCA known, pointed to an important role of serotonin in the induction of such effects.

Not surprisingly, most controlled (placebo-controlled, randomized trials often with comparator drug) studies on antidepressants have been performed by pharmaceutical companies during the initial phases of drug development. If such trials were specifically aimed for sexual side effects, often a comparator drug was included that either displayed considerable sexual side effects (an SSRI) or had a low sexual side effect profile, like bupropion [12], an antidepressant that blocks noradrenergic and dopaminergic (DA) reuptake sites without any effect on the serotonin transporter (SERT). In comparator antidepressant studies of SSRIs versus bupropion, the SSRIs always have a higher incidence of sexual complaints than bupropion. Coleman et al. [13] reported 30% sexual complaints on fluoxetine compared to 10% on bupropion in a placebo-controlled study. In a double-blind, placebo-controlled study on sertraline and bupropion in major depressed patients [14], sertraline induced far higher sexual complaints than bupropion (52% versus 8%). This was also found in studies on sertraline versus bupropion [15], paroxetine versus bupropion [16], escitalopram versus bupropion [17], and venlafaxine (a noradrenaline/serotonin reuptake blocker-SNRI) versus bupropion [18]. Recently, new SSRIs with additional serotonergic mechanisms like vilazodone and vortioxetine were introduced. Vilazodone, an SSRI with 5-HT_{1A} receptor agonistic effects, showed a low propensity to induce sexual dysfunction. Although a statistically significant decrease in libido was reported, no or minimal differences were reported in sexual side effects in pooled data from three randomized, double-blind, placebo-controlled studies in almost 500 depressed adult patients [19–21]. Vortioxetine is an SSRI that also exerts agonistic activity at 5-HT_{1A} and 5-HT_{1B} receptors and antagonistic activity at 5-HT_3, 5-HT_7, and 5-HT_{1D} receptors [22, 23]. Vortioxetine is an efficient antidepressant and has a low sexual side effect profile [21, 22]. The additional mechanisms in the mode of action of vilazodone (5-HT_{1A} agonist) and vortioxetine (5-$HT_{1A/1B}$ agonist and 5-$HT_{3/7/1D}$ antagonist) apparently antagonize the sexual inhibitory actions of the SSRI-moiety of the respective molecules. These additional mechanisms do not clearly jeopardize the antidepressant effects that probably are caused by the SSRI activity. This may lead to the hypothesis that the antidepressant effects and the sexual side effects induced by an SSRI are caused by different mechanisms in the brain that can be separately influenced by other (serotonergic) mechanisms and may lead to selective antagonizing of the sexual side effects. It is extremely difficult if not impossible to elucidate the exact underlying mechanisms of such complex acting antidepressants in humans. Combination of two (or more) separate drugs, e.g., an SSRI combined with reboxetine (a noradrenalin reuptake inhibitor-NRI) or bupropion a noradrenalin-dopamine reuptake inhibitor (NDRI) could lead to some answers but the combination is accompanied by several complicated interactions, not only at the level of side effects, but also at pharmacokinetic and metabolism levels. Such studies suffer always from complicated results that are often not clear-cut at all. Development of new antidepressants with less or no sexual side effects (as they appear the main reason for stopping treatment at long-term use) seems an important way to go.

The need for new and effective treatment of depression is clearly influenced by the need for less or milder side effects (not only sexual ones). Moreover, additional benefits like a fast onset of action of the antidepressant activity (days instead of weeks), a higher efficacy (present antidepressants are only working in 40–60% of the depressed patients), and a reasonable price may lead to new antidepressants that have enormous advantages over the existing "low cost" antidepressants (TCAs and SSRIs).

3. Translational studies into the putative sexual side effects of novel antidepressants

From all the human studies on antidepressants and sexual side effects, a strong pattern emerges: SSRIs, drugs that block serotonergic transporters at serotonergic neurons, have intrinsic effects on sexual behavior. Other antidepressants, like bupropion that lack serotonergic activity, have no or less sexual side effects and may even be beneficially in alleviating the often already lowered libido of depressed patients [24]. In the search for new and better antidepressants, an animal model with a high predictive validity for sexual (side) effects is an indispensable asset. It is of paramount importance that such an animal model should be as predictive as possible for the human (depressed) patient. An ideal animal model should follow the human course of the emergence of sexual side effects of present SSRIs: not acute, but after (sub) chronic administration. The emergence of the sexual side effects more or less parallels the emergence of the antidepressant activity that takes weeks to develop gradually. The animal model has also to be able to detect prosexual effects of drugs, as this may be an important factor in the treatment of either the SSRI-induced sexual dysfunctions or in the improvement of the basically lowered sexual drive (libido) associated with the depression itself. Ideally, the model should also be able to determine a fast(er) onset of action of new antidepressants, whereas long-term efficacy (years) is a must because antidepressant treatment lasts often for a very long time.

4. The actual animal model

Several years ago we noticed that upon testing of young adult male outbred (Wistar strain) rats on their sexual performance against a female rat brought into behavioral estrus, individual males exhibited variable levels of sexual activity. Some rats were sexually very active, some not at all and the rest with a variety of intermediate levels [25]. We standardly test all males subsequently for four weekly tests of 30 minutes, which generates very stable levels of sexual behavior in individual males. At the third to fourth test individual rats have a very stable and long-lasting level of sexual performance. The number of ejaculations per 30 min is a very reliable and predictive measure of the sexual performance of male rats and we hypothesized that male rats display sexual endophenotypes [26]. Over the last decade we tested (trained) more than 2000 male rats (of the Wistar outbred strain) in this way and we established that such rats might be distributed according to their sexual endophenotype [27, 28] in slow (sluggish), average (normal), and fast ejaculators. On average 20–30% of the rats are "slow" performers (0–1 ejaculation/30 min) and 10% are fast performers (4–5 ejaculations per 30 min). Animals with 2–3 ejaculations per test are regarded as "average" or normal ejaculators and constitute the bulk of all rats (60–70%). We hypothesized that male rats notoriously low in sexual performance might model delayed or retarded (an) ejaculation in human males, and those with four or more ejaculations per test reflecting premature ejaculation in men [26].

In the present contribution we focus on average ejaculating rats. They are ideally suited to test the effects of antidepressants or other psychotropic drugs on sexual behavior because both inhibitory and stimulatory (prosexual) properties can be detected.

To assess putative sexual side effects of psychotropic drugs we designed an experimental drug test consisting of 14 days of daily drug treatment followed by a week washout to judge the reversibility of a putative drug effect [28]. Sexual behavior is measured for 30 min after acute, sub-chronic (1 week), and chronic (2 weeks) treatment and a week after stopping treatment (washout).

Critical factors in using an animal model over time (years) are the reproducibility and stability of the model. Our standard control SSRI that we always used as positive control reference drug in our studies is paroxetine, an SSRI with rather severe sexual side effects in humans. We analyzed the effects of one dose of paroxetine (10 mg/kg p.o.) in seven subsequent experiments performed over several years using the protocol as described by Chan et al. [28]. After placing an estrus female into the cage of a sexually trained rat the male starts sniffing and following the female. Ensuing, the female responds by displaying the typical proceptive behaviors hopping and darting, upon which the male starts mounting and intromitting the female, finally leading to an ejaculation. Usually a series of mounts and intromissions occurs (introductory male sexual behavior) leading to the consummatory phase, ejaculation, which is followed by a rest period (postejaculatory interval) after which the male resumes the next series of mounts and intromissions and finally again ejaculation (**Figure 1**). Most males show around 2–3 ejaculations per 30 min, but this number may vary from 0 to 5 ejaculations.

Figure 2 shows the number of ejaculations per test (30 min) of sexually trained rats with an average ejaculation rate (2–3 ejaculations/30 min) after vehicle or paroxetine (10 mg/kg p.o.) treatment. The sexual behavior of all animals was measured acutely (30 min after administration), sub-chronically (after 1 week administration), chronically (after 2 weeks administration), and after washout (1 week after stopping treatment). Overall, the vehicle treated animals did not differ over tests (time) significantly in ejaculation frequency ($F_{18,171} = 1253$ n.s.) and latency to the first

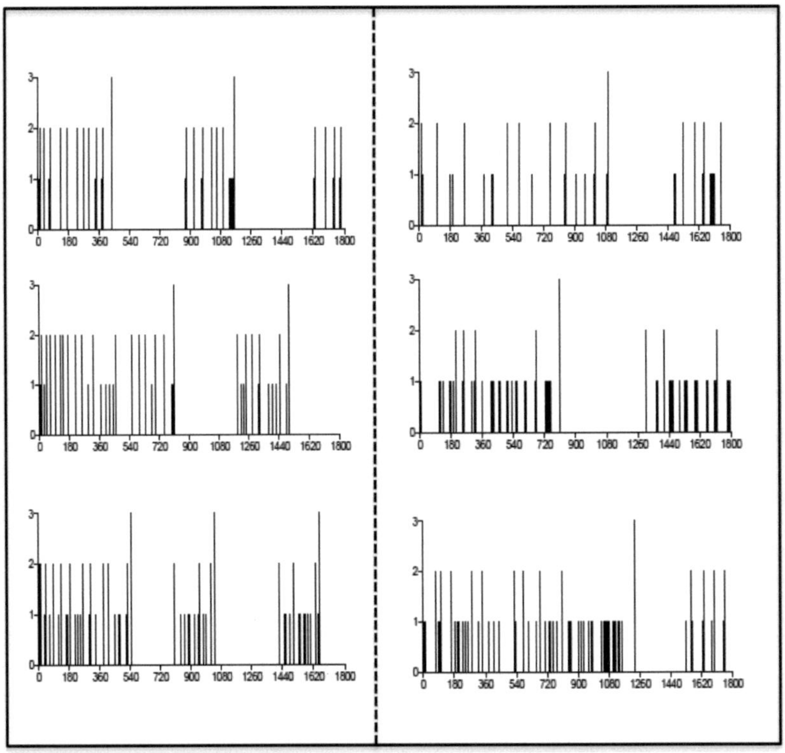

Figure 1. Representative examples of sexual behavior pattern of experienced male Wistar rats chronically treated with vehicle (left) or paroxetine (right) during a 30 min test with an estrus female. 1 = mount, 2 = intromission, 3 = ejaculation.

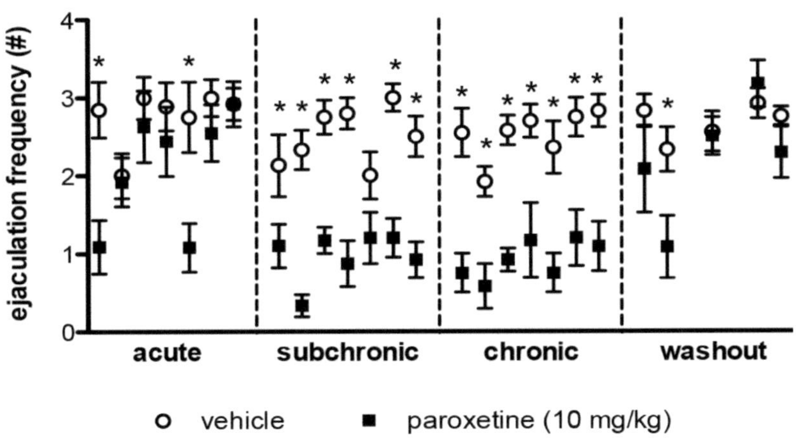

Figure 2. The ejaculation frequencies of seven cohorts of male rats tested against an estrus female rat during a 30 min test. The independent seven cohorts were tested over a time span of approx. 4 years. The data of the vehicle groups (open circles) and the paroxetine groups (10 mg/kg p.o.) are shown after acute, sub-chronic, and chronic treatment with either vehicle or paroxetine. One week after cessation of treatment a last sexual test was performed in order to study whether the sexual behavior returned to the original level. Asterisk (*) indicates significant difference between the vehicle and paroxetine group.

ejaculation ($F_{15,168}$ = 1360 n.s.) showing the stability of male sexual behavior across experiments and time. Paroxetine showed a very stable reduction in the number of ejaculation (**Figure 2**) and increase in the latency to ejaculate (not shown) after 1 and 2 weeks of administration compared to vehicle treatment. One week after cessation of treatment (washout) paroxetine pretreated groups returned to normal levels (in four of five experiments), and there were no differences between the acute treatment and the washout data.

These data confirm the reliability and stability of the paradigm used for measuring sexual behavior and drug effects. This allows the direct comparison of different psychotropic drugs tested in separate experiments.

5. Dose-dependency of drug effects on sexual behavior

Sexual side effects in humans are dose-dependent, although human studies often do not investigate several doses (dose-dependency) in one experiment. In general, higher doses of antidepressants lead to much more serious side effects, including sexual effects. Therefore, in our animal model we always tried to test increasing doses in order to possibly generate a dose-response curve. In case of paroxetine, doses of 2.5, 5, and 10 mg/kg (p.o.) were tested using our standard experimental design.

Figure 3 (left column; top figure) shows the results. Paroxetine acutely given did not affect the ejaculation frequency but showed a dose-dependent effect after sub-chronic and chronic administration, although the 5-mg/kg dose did not significantly differ from the highest dose (10 mg/kg). Although not shown here, other parameters measured (e.g., latency to ejaculation and post-ejaculatory latency) also showed the inhibitory profile of paroxetine. This pattern of paroxetine's inhibitory action in rat's sexual behavior parallels the human situation where at least 1 week of administration is needed to induce sexual dysfunctions [29, 30]. Looking into the structure of the sexual performance in rats, paroxetine changes the sexual behavior pattern after sub-chronic and chronic dosing. More mounts are needed to reach the same amount of intromissions, reflected in the increased intromission latency and increased mount frequency and the decreased copulatory efficiency. Rats show a decreased "hit rate," i.e., attempts to reach vaginal penetration. This is also evident in the increased ejaculation latency (for details see Table 1 and Figure 4 in [31]).

All SSRIs share the inhibitory action on male sexual behavior after (sub) chronic but not acute administration (**Table 1**). This pattern clearly follows the antidepressant profile which also emerges only after some delay after starting treatment. Apparently, the mechanisms underlying the inhibitory effects of SSRIs after repeated administration reflect changes in the serotonergic system which become manifest only after sustained administration. The underlying hypothesis, increased serotonin-mediated tonic inhibition, suggests that chronic SSRI treatment influences underlying circuitry mediating sexual behavior by enhancing 5-HT activity in projection areas [32]. Although it is not at all clear that how this mechanism specifically acts at various brain levels, it is evident that a very complex network in the brain and spinal cord is

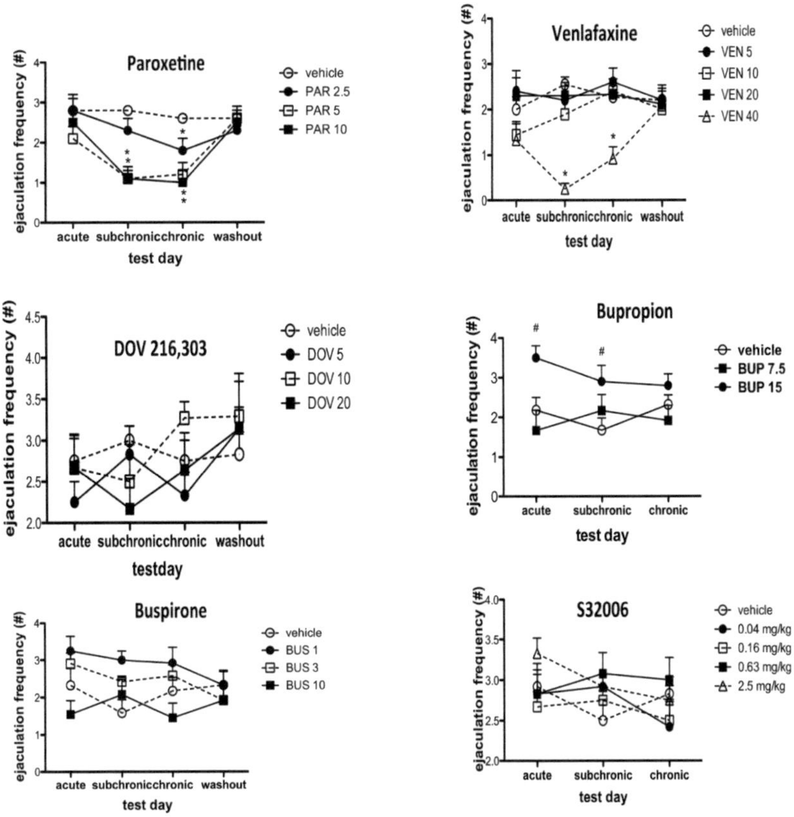

Figure 3. The effects of paroxetine (left, top), venlafaxine (right, top), DOV 216,303 (left, middle), bupropion (right, middle), buspirone (left, bottom), and S32006 (right, bottom) on the ejaculation frequency are shown after acute, subchronic, and chronic administration as well as after 1 week of washout.

involved in this serotonergically induced action, including important roles for noradrenergic, dopaminergic, and glutamatergic systems [33].

The serotonin-noradrenalin reuptake inhibitor (SNRI) venlafaxine affects male sexual behavior at relatively high doses (**Figure 3**, right column, top). Because noradrenaline exerts facilitatory effects in sexual behavior in humans [31], one might hypothetically expect that this may contrast the inhibitory effects of the SSRI-component in venlafaxine. Although at lower doses (that are antidepressant in animal depression models) venlafaxine does not affect sexual behavior, at the higher dose tested it does, indicating that the SSRI activity becomes dominant in venlafaxine's action.

The dopaminergic (DA) system plays an important role in the facilitation of sexual behavior [34]. DA activity in mesolimbic areas is involved in motivational and copulatory aspects of sexual behavior. There is a strong 5-HT/DA interaction in the brain, which modulates motivational aspects of sexual performance [31] and adding a dopaminergic stimulating mechanism to an inhibiting serotonergic mechanism (e.g., SSRI) might result in amelioration of the inhibitory action of the latter [31]. DOV 216,303 is a triple monoaminergic reuptake inhibitor (TRI) that blocks noradrenergic, serotonergic, and dopaminergic transporters [35, 36].

One of the core symptoms of depression, anhedonia, is connected to a lowered mesolimbic DA neurotransmission and the original rationale for development of TRIs was to alleviate anhedonia in depression [36]. An additional advantage might be that the dopaminergic stimulation by DA-reuptake inhibition might reverse sexual side effects. No data are available on the sexual side effect profile of TRIs, but a recent trial with a TRI (the DOV 216,303 isomer amitifadine) showed no worsening of sexual functioning after chronic treatment of depressed patients [37]. The preclinical data (**Figure 3** left column, middle) confirm the lack of sexual side effects of DOV 216,303 at doses that exert antidepressant effects in animal models of depression [36, 38–40]. This clearly suggests that 5-HT mediated inhibition of sexual behavior can be overcome by stimulating dopaminergic neurotransmission via dopamine transporter (DAT)-blockade, although a role for noradrenaline cannot be excluded.

Bupropion is well known for its counteractive effects on SSRI-induced sexual dysfunctions [17]. Bupropion facilitates noradrenergic and dopaminergic mechanisms (it is a noradrenalin transporter(NET) and DAT antagonist) and we expected a rather strong prosexual effect of bupropion in our animal model. Bupropion had a slight stimulating effect on sexual behavior, but only at the higher dose and only after acute and (marginally) sub-chronic dosing, but not at chronic administration (**Figure 3**, right column; middle). This small and short-living facilitatory effect of bupropion was rather unexpected. Apomorphine [41], a mixed dopamine D_2/D_3 receptor agonist showed a comparable profile in a similar experiment (**Table 1**),

Drug	Mechanism of action	Acute	Sub-chronic	Chronic	Washout	Reference
Paroxetine	SSRI	0	↓	↓	0	[31]
Fluvoxamine	SSRI	0	0	↓	nt	[59]
Citalopram	SSRI	0 (↓)	↓	↓	0	[57, 60]
Fluoxetine	SSRI	0	↓	↓	nt	[61]
Venlafaxine	SNRI	0	0	↓	0	[31]
Bupropion	NDRI	↑	0	0	0	[31]
DOV 216,303	TRI	0	0	↓	0	[31]
Buspirone	5-HT_{1A} R Agonist	↑	0	0	0	[31]
Vilazodone	SSRI/5-HT_{1A} R agonist	0	0	0	0	[56, 57]
Vortioxetine	SSRI/$5\text{-HT}_{1A,1B}$ R agonist; $5\text{-HT}_{3,7,1D}$ R antagonist	0	0	0	0	[58]
Tramadol	SNRI/μ-opioid R agonist	0↓	nt	nt	nt	[62]
Apomorphine	DA-$D_{2/3}$ R agonist	↑	↑	↑	nt	[41]
S32006	5-HT_{2C} R antagonist	0	0	0	0	[31]
WAY100,635	5-HT_{1A} R antagonist	0	0	0	nt	[60]

↓: inhibition; ↑: stimulation; 0: no effect; nt: not tested. SSRI. selective serotonergic reuptake inhibitor; SNRI: serotonergic and noradrenergic reuptake inhibitor; NDRI: noradrenergic and dopaminergic reuptake inhibitor; TRI: triple monoaminergic reuptake inhibitor; R: receptor.

Table 1. Summary of effects of various drugs on male sexual behavior after acute, sub-chronic, or chronic treatment.

although it had a somewhat stronger prosexual effect than bupropion. Apparently, the relatively weak DAT-blockade of bupropion might be not strong enough to permanently stimulate sexual behavior in healthy subjects (like our rats), leaving open the possibility that in "depressed" brains with an extra SSRI-induced sexual dysfunction, bupropion might be very effective as an "add-on" medication. We have not tried bupropion in our SSRI (paroxetine)-treated model as an add-on yet.

When an SSRI is given (either to man or animal) the pharmacological mechanism, blockade of the SERT on the neuron induces an increase in the level of 5-HT in the synaptic cleft [42]. 5-HT is the endogenous ligand of all 14 different 5-HT receptors and it is very likely that some but not all 5-HT receptors are involved in serotonin's action in sexual behavior. One of the receptors involved is the 5-HT_{1A} receptor, located as a somatodendritic autoreceptor on 5-HT cell bodies and as postsynaptic heteroreceptor on many nonserotonergic neurons in various brain areas [42]. 5-HT_{1A} receptor agonists including buspirone have prosexual activity in rats upon acute administration [43, 44]. Extensive evidence suggests that this prosexual activity of 5-HT_{1A} R agonists is most likely due to activation of postsynaptic 5-HT_{1A} receptors that probably mediate dopaminergic activation in brain areas that decrease the ejaculation threshold [44]. Clinically, the only available (partial) 5-HT_{1A} receptor agonist buspirone (also a dopamine D_2 receptor antagonist) is used as an antidepressant and has not been associated with sexual side effects [45, 46]. In our model in rats, low doses of buspirone which are also exerting antidepressant effects in animal depression models have mild prosexual activity (**Figure 3** left column; lower panel). Our rat data are in line with (limited) human data which indicate that buspirone does not exert sexual side effects as well as it is not a very strong add-on drug in combination with SSRIs. The absence of prosexual effects at the highest dose could reveal the dopamine D_2 receptor blocking activity of buspirone which certainly comes in action at this dose. Dopamine D_2 receptor blockade has strong inhibitory effects on sexual behavior and interferes at higher doses with the prosexual activity of the 5-HT_{1A} receptor stimulation.

We have tested a selective 5-HT_{2C} receptor antagonist (S32006) in our rat model (**Figure 3**, right column; bottom panel). 5-HT_{2C} receptor agonists induce penile erections in rats and facilitate ejaculation via 5-HT_{2C} receptor activation in the lumbosacral spinal cord [47, 48]. Because 5-HT_{2C} receptor activation by d-LSD and quipazine induce increased ejaculation latencies, it has been suggested that the inhibition pattern by SSRIs has resemblance to that of 5-HT_{2C} receptor activation [49]. Novel nonSSRI antidepressants like agomelatine and mirtazapine lack sexual side effects [50]. Augmentation therapy with mirtazapine seems to decrease the sexual side effects of SSRIs [51, 52] supporting the notion of SSRI-induced sexual dysfunction mediated via 5-HT_{2C} receptors. S32006 is a very selective 5-HT_{2C} receptor antagonist, has antidepressant effects in preclinical depression models and elevates extracellular DA and NA, but not 5-HT [53, 54]. S32006 was completely devoid of any effect on sexual behavior after acute, sub-chronic and chronic administration [31], suggesting that 5-HT_{2C} receptors are not (directly) involved in sexual effects induced by SSRIs.

Recently, some new antidepressants were introduced in the market, vilazodone and vortioxetine. Vilazodone is an SSRI and a partial 5-HT_{1A} receptor agonist that has antidepressant activity in man and rat. Although much more clinical research is needed, the initial clinical trials suggested the absence of (additional) sexual side effects during treatment of the depressed patients [55].

We tested vilazodone (1, 3, and 10 mg/kg p.o.) and as reference drugs citalopram (10 and 30 mg/kg p.o.) and paroxetine (10 mg/kg p.o.) in our standard rat model [56]. Vilazodone did not affect sexual behavior at any dose or after acute, sub-chronic, or chronic administration, whereas both citalopram and paroxetine showed the typical SSRI profile: no acute effects but inhibitory effects at sub-chronic and chronic administration. In a subsequent experiment [57] once daily paroxetine (10 mg/kg p.o.), vilazodone (10 mg/kg p.o.), paroxetine (10 mg/kg p.o.) plus buspirone (3 mg/kg p.o.) or vehicle were given for 14 days to male rats and then switched for 7 days to various treatments. Vehicle, paroxetine, and vilazodone pretreated groups were switched to vehicle; paroxetine pretreated groups were switched to vilazodone, paroxetine plus buspirone or vehicle and the paroxetine plus buspirone group was switched to paroxetine alone. Sexual behavior was scored acutely (1 h after dosing), after 7 days dosing and after 14 days dosing as well as after 7 days after switching. The combination of paroxetine plus buspirone, like vilazodone alone, did not have an effect on sexual behavior, while paroxetine alone reduced it considerably. Switching to paroxetine in both the paroxetine plus buspirone group as well as in the vilazodone group resulted in clear sexual inhibitory effects. These studies strongly suggest that the 5-HT_{1A} receptor agonistic activity in the vilazodone molecule counteracts the inhibitory action of the SSRI part. These preclinical data strongly support the clinical studies that suggest absence of sexual side effects due to the antidepressant. The findings also suggest that adding a 5-HT_{1A} receptor agonist (like buspirone) to an SSRI may indeed counteract the SSRI-induced sexual dysfunctions.

Another recently developed and introduced antidepressant, vortioxetine, is an SSRI with an additional complex profile. Next to inhibiting the SERT, it exerts agonistic activity at 5-HT_{1A} and 5-HT_{1B} receptors and antagonistic activity at 5-HT_{3}, 5-HT_{7}, and 5-HT_{1D} receptors [22].

Vortioxetine (1 and 10 mg/kg, p.o.) did not affect sexual behavior in male rats, neither after acute, sub-chronic, and chronic dosing [58]. The doses used led to, respectively, 50% (1 mg/kg) and 90% (10 mg/kg) SERT occupation. In the same experiment, the reference paroxetine (at 10 mg/kg) had a comparable SERT occupancy of 90% as the highest vortioxetine dose, indicative that at least at the highest dose tested vortioxetine showed sufficient SERT occupancy to induce sexual side effects. It is therefore clear that the remaining mechanisms in vortioxetine ($5\text{-HT}_{3,7,1A,1B,1D}$) in some as yet not understood way counteract the SSRI-induced inhibitory effects. Ongoing research tries to further unravel this mechanism. Based on our finding in rats, vortioxetine is predicted being devoid of (extra) sexual side effects in depressed patients. Clinical findings, although not explicitly aimed to study the sexual side effects of vortioxetine (e.g., in healthy people), indeed hint to a low propensity of vortioxetine in this area [22].

6. Discussion

Serotonin is critically involved in the mechanisms underlying various aspects of sexual behavior, both in men and male rats. Nowadays, the main treatment of depression uses SSRIs. They are strongly associated with sexual side effects that frequently lead to stopping the antidepressant treatment. SSRIs increase the serotonergic tone in the central nervous system, leading to a cascade, although largely unknown, of neurochemical changes that in some way or another lead to sexual dysfunctions, in particular, after longer (weeks) treatment. The antidepressant quality of SSRIs is generally considered as reasonable whereas other side effects of SSRIs (like dizziness, nausea) are tolerable and disappear upon continuous treatment. The sexual side effects do not disappear and are troublesome. Thus, there is a great need to get rid of these effects and newly developed antidepressants are scrutinized for their induction of sexual dysfunction. Recently, two new antidepressants, vilazodone and vortioxetine have been introduced and both compounds claim a low propensity to induce sexual side effects. Both compounds have an important SSRI function in their mechanism of action that more or less guarantees antidepressant effects, and also have additional inherent pharmacological mechanisms that presumably antagonize the inhibitory sexual effects caused by the SSRI mechanism. The clinical use of both drugs over the coming years will further elucidate their propensity to induce sexual side effects.

Over the last decade, we have developed a male rat sexual behavior paradigm that models to a large extent the human situation. Classic SSRIs (fluoxetine, paroxetine, fluvoxamine, citalopram, escitalopram, sertraline) have sexual behavior inhibiting effects, not after acute but after (sub) chronic administration. This mimics the human situation where such effects emerge after longer (weeks) administration and do not disappear upon continuous use (months, years), which is also the case in our rat model. Some compounds (e.g., buspirone, bupropion) are active after acute administration. Whether this is also the case in humans is unknown because of lack of studies. Our model is also fit to measure the effects of psychotropics in addition to antidepressants. We have studied various drugs, e.g., apomorphine, tramadol [62], and several serotonergic drugs and have found inhibitory, facilitatory, or no effects. The model is very useful to study the brain mechanisms underlying various aspects of sexual behavior and of sexual dysfunction. The most remarkable characteristics of the model are its reliability and reproducibility. Each male rat appears to have an endophenotype with regard to its sexual behavior that becomes very stable after a number of sexual training sessions. Whether such sexual endophenotypes are present in men is unclear but the presence of lifelong premature ejaculation suggests that possibility. It is at least clear that much more research is needed to unravel such hypotheses in humans.

7. Conclusion

Sexual side effects are a major concern in presently used antidepressants, especially the SSRIs. Several strategies have been used to circumvent these problems but are rather disappointing. Newly developed antidepressants like vortioxetine and vilazodone seem to be devoid of sexual side effects in humans, although large scale data are not yet available. In the search for new antidepressants that lack sexual side effects, animal models can play an important role. A rat model of sexual (dys)function is illustrated, which seems to fulfill the face, predictive, and construct validities for a valuable animal model. The model can also be used to investigate underlying mechanisms in the control of sexual functions and dysfunctions.

Author details

Jocelien D.A. Olivier[1], Diana C. Esquivel Franco[1], Marcel D. Waldinger[2] and Berend Olivier[1,3,4]*

*Address all correspondence to: b.olivier@uu.nl

1 Groningen Institute for Evolutionary Life Sciences, Faculty of Science and Engineering, Rijksuniversiteit Groningen, Groningen, The Netherlands

2 Department of Pharmacology and Physiology, Drexell University College of Medicine, Philadelphia, USA

3 Department of Psychopharmacology, Science Faculty, Utrecht University, Utrecht, The Netherlands

4 Department of Psychiatry, Yale University School of Medicine, New Haven, USA

References

[1] Pfaus JG. Pathways of sexual desire. The Journal of Sexual Medicine. 2009;**6**:1506-1533. DOI: 10.1111/j.1743-6109.2009.01309.x

[2] Makhlouf A, Kparker A, Niederberger CS. Depression and erectile dysfunction. The Urologic Clinics of North America. 2007;**34**:565-574

[3] Higgins A, Nash M, Lynch AM. Antidepressant-associated sexual dysfunction: Impact, effects, and treatment. Drug Health Patient Safety. 2010;**2**:141-150. DOI: 10.2147/DHPS.S7634

[4] Lahon K, Shetty HM, Paramel A, Sharma G. Sexual dysfunction with the use of antidepressants in a tertiary care mental health setting—A retrospective case series. The Journal of Pharmacology & Pharmacotherapeutics. 2011;**2**:128-131. DOI: 10.4103/0976-500X.81913

[5] Monteiro WO, Noshirvani HF, Marks IM, Lelliott PT. Anorgasmia from clomipramine in obsessive-compulsive disorder. A controlled trial. The British Journal of Psychiatry. 1987;**151**:107-112

[6] Beaumont G. Sexual side-effects of clomipramine (Anafranil). The Journal of International Medical Research. 1977;**5**:37-44

[7] Balon R. Depression, antidepressants and human sexuality. Primary Psychiatry. 2007;**14**: 42-50

[8] Segraves RT. Sexual dysfunction associated with antidepressant therapy. The Urologic clinics of North America. 2007;**34**:575-579

[9] Segraves RT, Balon R. Antidepressant-induced sexual dysfunction in men. Pharmacology, Biochemistry and Behavior. 2014;**121**:132-137. DOI: 10.1016/j.pbb.2013.11.003

[10] Montejo-González AL, Llorca G, Izquierdo JA, Ledesma A, Bousoño M, Calcedo A, Carrasco JL, Ciudad J, Daniel E, De la Gandara J, Derecho J, Franco M, Gomez MJ, Macias JA, Martin T, Perez V, Sanchez JM, Sanchez S, Vicens E. SSRI-induced sexual dysfunction: Fluoxetine, paroxetine, sertraline, and fluvoxamine in a prospective, multicenter, and descriptive clinical study of 344 patients. Journal of Sex & Marital Therapy. 1997;**23**:176-194

[11] Harrison WM, Rabkin JG, Ehrhardt AA, Stewart JW, McGrath PJ, Ross D, Quitkin FM. Effects of antidepressant medication on sexual function: A controlled study. Journal of Clinical Psychopharmacology. 1986;**6**:144-149

[12] Latorre A, Guipponi G, Duffy D, Conca A. Sexual dysfunction related to psychoptropic drugs: A critical review-part 1: Antidepressants. Pharmacopsychiatry. 2013;**46**:191-199

[13] Coleman CC1, King BR, Bolden-Watson C, Book MJ, Segraves RT, Richard N, Ascher J, Batey S, Jamerson B, Metz A. A placebo-controlled comparison of the effects on sexual functioning of bupropion sustained release and fluoxetine. Clinical Therapeutics. 2001;**23**:1040-1058

[14] Segraves RT, Kavoussi R, Hughes AR, Batey SR, Johnston JA, Donahue R, Ascher JA. Evaluation of sexual functioning in depressed outpatients: A double-blind comparison of sustained-release bupropion and sertraline treatment. Journal of Clinical Psychopharmacology. 2000;**20**:122-128

[15] Croft H, Settle E Jr, Houser T, Batey SR, Donahue RM, Ascher JA. A placebo-controlled comparison of the antidepressant efficacy and effects on sexual functioning of sustained-release bupropion and sertraline. Clinical Therapeutics. 1999;**21**:643-658

[16] Kennedy SH, Fulton KA, Bagby RM, Greene AL, Cohen NL, Rafi-Tari S. Sexual function during bupropion or paroxetine treatment of major depressive disorder. The Canadian Journal of Psychiatry. 2006;**51**:234-242

[17] Clayton AH, Croft HA, Horrigan JP, Wightman DS, Krishen A, Richard NE, Modell JG. Bupropion extended release compared with escitalopram: Effects on sexual functioning and antidepressant efficacy in 2 randomized, double-blind, placebo-controlled studies. The Journal of Clinical Psychiatry. 2006;**67**:736-746

[18] Thase ME, Clayton AH, Haight BR, Thompson AH, Modell JG, Johnston JA. A double-blind comparison between bupropion XL and venlafaxine XR: Sexual functioning, antidepressant efficacy, and tolerability. Journal of Clinical Psychopharmacology. 2006;**26**:482-488

[19] Khan A, Cutler AJ, Kajdasz DK, Gallipoli S, Athanasiou M, Robinson DS, Whalen H, Reed CR. A randomized, double-blind, placebo-controlled, 8-week study of vilazodone, a serotonergic agent for the treatment of major depressive disorder. The Journal of Clinical Psychiatry. 2011;**72**:441-447. DOI: 10.4088/JCP.10m06596

[20] Clayton AH, Kennedy SH, Edwards JB, Gallipoli S, Reed CR. The effect of vilazodone on sexual function during the treatment of major depressive disorder. The Journal of Sexual Medicine. 2013;**10**:2465-2476. DOI: 10.1111/jsm.12004

[21] Deardorff WJ, Grossberg GT. A review of the clinical efficacy, safety and tolerability of the antidepressants vilazodone, levomilnacipran and vortioxetine. Expert Opinion on Pharmacotherapy. 2014;**15**:25-42. DOI: 10.1517/14656566.2014.960842

[22] Sanchez C, Asin KE, Artigas F. Vortioxetine, a novel antidepressant with multi-modal activity: Review of preclinical and clinical data. Pharmacology & Therapeutics. 2015;**145**:43-57. DOI: 10.1016/j.pharmthera.2014.07.001

[23] Gibb AI, Deeks ED. Vortioxetine: First global approval. Drugs. 2014;**74**:135-145. DOI: 10.1007/s40265-013-0161-9

[24] Dorevitch A, Davis H. Fluvoxamine-associated sexual dysfunction. The Annals of pharmacotherapy. 1994;**28**:872-874

[25] Pattij T, de Jong TR, Uitterdijk A, Waldinger MD, Veening JG, Cools AR, van der Graaf PH, Olivier B. Individual differences in male rat ejaculatory behaviour: Searching for models to study ejaculation disorders. The European Journal of Neuroscience. 2005;**22**:724-734

[26] Olivier B, Chan JS, Pattij T, de Jong TR, Oosting RS, Veening JG, Waldinger MD. Psychopharmacology of male rat sexual behavior: Modeling human sexual dysfunctions?. International Journal of Impotence Research. 2006;**18**(1):423

[27] Chan JS, Olivier B, de Jong TR, Snoeren EM, Kooijman E, van Hasselt FN, Limpens JH, Kas MJ, Waldinger MD, Oosting RS. Translational research into sexual disorders: pharmacology and genomics. European Journal of Pharmacology. 2008;**585**:426-435. DOI: 10.1016/j.ejphar.2008.02.098

[28] Chan JS, Waldinger MD, Olivier B, Oosting RS. Drug-induced sexual dysfunction in rats. Current Protocols in Neuroscience. 2010;**Chapter 9**:Unit 9.34. DOI: 10.1002/0471142301.ns0934s53

[29] Balon R. Modifications of the serotonin system by antidepressant treatments: Implications for the therapeutic response in major depression. The American Journal of Psychiatry. 2006;**163**:1504-1509

[30] Waldinger MD, Zwinderman AH, Olivier B. SSRIs and ejaculation: A double-blind, randomized, fixed-dose study with paroxetine and citalopram. Journal of Clinical Psychopharmacology. 2001;**21**:556-560

[31] Bijlsma EY, Chan JS, Olivier B, Veening JG, Millan MJ, Waldinger MD, Oosting RS. Sexual side effects of serotonergic antidepressants: Mediated by inhibition of serotonin on central dopamine release? Pharmacology, Biochemistry and Behavior. 2014,**121**.88-101. DOI: 10.1016/j.pbb.2013.10.004

[32] Blier P, de Montigny C, Chaput Y. Modifications of the serotonin system by antidepressant treatments. Implications for the therapeutic response in major depression. Journal of Clinical Psychopharmacology. 1987;**7**(6 Suppl):24S-35S

[33] Will RG, Hull M, Dominguez JM. Influences of dopamine and glutamate in the medial preoptic area on male sexual behavior. Pharmacology Biochemistry & Behavior. 2014; **121**:115-123. DOI: 10.1016/j.pbb.2014.02.005

[34] Hull EM, Muschamp JW, Sato S. Dopamine and serotonin: Influences on male sexual behavior. Physiology & Behavior. 2004;**83**:291-307

[35] Skolnick P, Popik P, Janowsky A, Beer B, Lippa AS. Antidepressant-like actions of DOV 21,947: A "triple" reuptake inhibitor. European Journal of Pharmacology. 2003;**461**:99-104

[36] Skolnick P, Krieter P, Tizzano J, Basile A, Popik P, Czobor P, Lippa A. Preclinical and clinical pharmacology of DOV 216,303, a "triple" reuptake inhibitor. CNS Drug Reviews. 2006;**12**:123-134

[37] Tran PI, Skolnick P, Czobor P, Huang NY, Bradshaw M, McKinney A, Fava M. Efficacy and tolerability of the novel triple reuptake inhibitor amitifadine in the treatment of patients with major depressive disorder: A randomized, double-blind, placebo-controlled trial. Journal of Psychiatric Research. 2012;**46**:64-71. DOI: 10.1016/j.jpsychires.2011.09.003

[38] Breuer ME, Chan JS, Oosting RS, Groenink L, Korte SM, Campbell U, Schreiber R, Hanania T, Snoeren EM, Waldinger M, Olivier B. The triple monoaminergic reuptake inhibitor DOV 216,303 has antidepressant effects in the rat olfactory bulbectomy model and lacks sexual side effects. European Neuropsychopharmacology. 2008;**18**:908-916. DOI: 10.1016/j.euroneuro.2008.07.011

[39] Caldarone BJ1, Paterson NE, Zhou J, Brunner D, Kozikowski AP, Westphal KG, Korte-Bouws GA, Prins J, Korte SM, Olivier B, Ghavami AJ. The novel triple reuptake inhibitor JZAD-IV-22 exhibits an antidepressant pharmacological profile without locomotor stimulant or sensitization properties. Journal of Pharmacology and Experimental Therapeutics. 2010;**335**:762-770. DOI: 10.1124/jpet.110.174011

[40] Paterson NE, Balci F, Campbell U, Olivier BE, Hanania T. The triple reuptake inhibitor DOV216,303 exhibits limited antidepressant-like properties in the differential reinforcement of low-rate 72-second responding assay, likely due to dopamine reuptake inhibition. Journal of Psychopharmacology. 2011;**25**:1357-1364. DOI: 10.1177/0269881110364272

[41] Olivier JD, de Jong TR, Jos Dederen P, van Oorschot R, Heeren D, Pattij T, Waldinger MD, Coolen LM, Cools AR, Olivier B, Veening JG. Effects of acute and chronic apomorphine on sex behavior and copulation-induced neural activation in the male rat. European Journal of Pharmacology. 2007;**576**:61-76

[42] Olivier B. Serotonin: A never-ending story. European Journal of Pharmacology. 2015;**753**: 2-18. DOI: 10.1016/j.ejphar.2014.10.031

[43] Åhlenius S, Larsson K, Svensson L, Hjorth S, Carlsson A, Lindberg P, Wikström H, Sanchez D, Arvidsson LE, Hacksell U, Nilsson JL. Effects of a new type of 5-HT receptor agonist on male rat sexual behavior. Pharmacology, Biochemistry and Behavior. 1981;**15**:785-792

[44] Snoeren EM, Veening JG, Olivier B, Oosting RS. Serotonin 1A receptors and sexual behavior in female rats: A review. Pharmacology, Biochemistry and Behavior. 2014;**121**:43-52. DOI: 10.1016/j.pbb.2013.11.017

[45] Landén M, Eriksson E, Agren H, Fahlén T. Effect of buspirone on sexual dysfunction in depressed patients treated with selective serotonin reuptake inhibitors. Journal of Clinical Psychopharmacology. 1999;**19**:268-271

[46] Landén M, Högberg P, Thase ME. Incidence of sexual side effects in refractory depression during treatment with citalopram or paroxetine. The Journal of Clinical Psychiatry. 2005;**66**:100-106

[47] Stafford SA, Tang K, Coote JH. Activation of lumbosacral 5-HT2C receptors induces bursts of rhythmic activity in sympathetic nerves to the vas deferens in male rats. British Journal of Pharmacology. 2006;**148**:1083-1090

[48] Yonezawa A, Yoshizumi M, Ebiko M, Ise SN, Watanabe C, Mizoguchi H, Kimura Y, Sakurada S. Ejaculatory response induced by a 5-HT2 receptor agonist m-CPP in rats: Differential roles of 5-HT2 receptor subtypes. Pharmacology, Biochemistry and Behavior. 2008;**88**:367-373

[49] Waldinger MD, Olivier B. Selective serotonin reuptake inhibitor-induced sexual dysfunction: Clinical and research considerations. International Clinical Psychopharmacology. 1998;**13**(Suppl 6):S27-33

[50] Millan MJ. Multi-target strategies for the improved treatment of depressive states: Conceptual foundations and neuronal substrates, drug discovery and therapeutic application. Pharmacology & Therapeutics. 2006;**110**:135-370

[51] Atmaca M, Korkmaz S, Topuz M, Mermi O. Mirtazapine augmentation for selective serotonin reuptake inhibitor-induced sexual dysfunction: A retrospective investigation. Psychiatry Investigation. 2011;**8**:55-57. DOI: 10.4306/pi.2011.8.1.55

[52] Ozmenler NK, Karlidere T, Bozkurt A, Yetkin S, Doruk A, Sutcigil L, Cansever A, Uzun O, Ozgen F, Ozsahin A. Mirtazapine augmentation in depressed patients with sexual dysfunction due to selective serotonin reuptake inhibitors. Human Psychopharmacology. 2008;**23**:321-326. DOI: 10.1002/hup.929

[53] Dekeyne A, Mannoury la Cour C, Gobert A, Brocco M, Lejeune F, Serres F, Sharp T, Daszuta A, Soumier A, Papp M, Rivet JM, Flik G, Cremers TI, Muller O, Lavielle G, Millan MJ. S32006, a novel 5-HT2C receptor antagonist displaying broad-based antidepressant and anxiolytic properties in rodent models. Psychopharmacology (Berlin). 2008;**199**:549-568. DOI: 10.1007/s00213-008-1177-9

[54] Millan MJ1, Brocco M, Gobert A, Dekeyne A. Anxiolytic properties of agomelatine, an antidepressant with melatoninergic and serotonergic properties: Role of 5-HT_{2C} receptor blockade. Psychopharmacology (Berlin). 2005;**177**:448-458

[55] Clayton AH, Gommoll C, Chen D, Nunez R, Mathews M. Sexual dysfunction during treatment of major depressive disorder with vilazodone, citalopram, or placebo: Results from a phase IV clinical trial. International Clinical Psychopharmacology. 2015;**30**:216-223. DOI: 10.1097/YIC.0000000000000075

[56] Oosting RS, Chan JS, Olivier B, Banerjee P. Vilazodone does not inhibit sexual behavior in male rats in contrast to paroxetine: A role for 5-HT1A receptors? Neuropharmacology. 2016;**107**:271-277. DOI: 10.1016/j.neuropharm.2016.03.045

[57] Oosting RS, Chan JS, Olivier B, Banerjee P, Choi YK, Tarazi F. Differential effects of vilazodone versus citalopram and paroxetine on sexual behaviors and serotonin transporter and receptors in male rats. Psychopharmacology (Berlin). 2016;**233**:1025-34. DOI: 10.1007/s00213-015-4198-1

[58] Li Y, Pehrson AL, Oosting RS, Gulinello M, Olivier B, Sanchez C. A study on time-and sex-dependent effects of vortioxetine on rat sexual behavior: possible role of direct receptor modulation. Neuropharmacology. 2017;**121**:89-99. DOI:10.1016/j.neuropharm.2017.04.017

[59] de Jong TR, Pattij T, Veening JG, Waldinger MD, Cools AR, Olivier B. Effects of chronic selective serotonin reuptake inhibitors on 8-OH-DPAT-induced facilitation of ejaculation in rats: Comparison of fluvoxamine and paroxetine. Psychopharmacology (Berlin). 2005;**179**:509-515

[60] de Jong TR, Pattij T, Veening JG, Dederen PJ, Waldinger MD, Cools AR, Olivier B. Citalopram combined with WAY 100635 inhibits ejaculation and ejaculation-related Fos immunoreactivity. European Journal of Pharmacology. 2005;**509**:49-59

[61] Vega Matuszczyk JI, Larsson K, Eriksson E. The selective serotonin reuptake inhibitor fluoxetine reduces sexual motivation in male rats. Pharmacology, Biochemistry and Behavior. 1998;**60**:527-32

[62] Olivier JDA, Esquivel Franco DC, Oosting RS, Waldinger MD, Sarnyai Z, Olivier B. Tramadol: Effects on sexual behavior in male rats are mainly caused by its 5-HT reuptake blocking effects. Neuropharmacology. 2017;**116**:50-58. DOI: 10.1016/j.neuropharm.2016.11.020

Section 5

Circumcision and Sexual (Dys)function

Chapter 5

A "Snip" in Time: Circumcision Revisited

Götz Egloff

Additional information is available at the end of the chapter

http://dx.doi.org/10.5772/intechopen.69106

Abstract

The publication of an Italian study on etiology and interactions of frenulum breve, frenulectomy, and premature ejaculation, and the results of a popular Austrian sex study initiated a survey on this topic, accompanied by collecting a small sample of data in an urban practice environment in Germany. Since frenulectomy, for practical reasons, often leads to a complete removal of the prepuce, circumcision has come to the fore anew. Moreover, under the heading, "Ending a myth: male circumcision is not associated with higher prevalence of erectile dysfunction," a recent study relating circumcision to sexual dysfunction has been published. In this chapter, an overview of research results as well as of psychological and clinical aspects of circumcision and associated subjects is given. There seem to be advantages of circumcision as to sexual dysfunction and premature ejaculation. Depending on etiopathology, some treatment options may require psychosomatic reasoning.

Keywords: sexual dysfunction, premature ejaculation, circumcision, psychosomatics, psychotherapy

1. Introduction and overview

While in northern European countries circumcision in males has no great tradition, the publication of an Italian study on etiology and interactions of frenulum breve, frenulectomy, and premature ejaculation (PE) [1] and the results of the popular 2011 Styrian Sex Study in Austria [2] initiated a survey on this topic, accompanied by collecting a small sample of data in an urban practice environment in Germany. The Styrian Sex Study of 2011 (n = 413) revealed high interest of Austrian male adolescents in circumcision, yet only 62% felt generally well informed (213). The Italian study at the Urological Department of Napoli University found a short frenulum (frenulum breve) that was treated by frenulectomy in 43% (59; n = 137) of patients with diagnosed PE. The authors observed diminishing of PE, and suggested that the treatment of premature ejaculation with frenulectomy could be used as first-line option. Since frenulectomy, for practical reasons, in practice often leads to a complete removal of the prepuce, a debate of this issue in the public has started which is long overdue. Moreover, under the heading, "Ending a myth: male circumcision is not associated with higher prevalence of erectile dysfunction" [3], a German study has officially confirmed what nobody in the field would seriously have put at question. In the study, rather a slight inverse significant correlation of satisfaction with erectile rigidity in circumcised men has been observed.

Sexual dysfunction issues are delicate issues, mostly multifactorial, and often associated with biographic aspects. Apart from vascular, neurological, and hormonal disorders (cf. [4]), etiology often involves psychosomatic factors. Psychogenic etiology has been implicated extensively; it can be traced back to Freud and his beginnings [5]. The differentiation between generalized and situational symptom formation has become highly important, since it points to biographical and relational aspects of which not only the latter have interactional functions. In practice more usual in female patients [6], who tend to relate dysfunction to their experiencing more often than males, psychosomatic sexual dysfunction can often be alleviated by psychotherapy. Moreover, the interconnections of hormones and psyche in females have been extensively explored [7], which has made psychosomatic reasoning of some dysfunction easier. This is not so much the case in somatogenic sexual dysfunction. Still, psyche is often involved in etiology, and it depends on etiology how to intervene. While in male sexual dysfunction often effective PDE-5 inhibitors [8, 9] aim at somatic functioning, which is an intervention in its own right, they also have psychosomatic impact. This will be discussed in the subsequent text.

Psychotherapeutic interventions are helpful in many psychic disorders, which is true for psychogenic sexual dysfunction, too. At any rate, from a psychoanalytic point of view, there is not only a necessity of getting grip on the psychodynamics of a patient's disorder in order to find an adequate intervention but, from a general point of view, also a necessity of understanding why, for example, some measures are or are not taken by patients. Even when something seems the obvious thing to do, their personalities, attitudes, and cultural predispositions may or may not keep them from doing so. Certainly, this is not to say what the right thing to do is.

Psychosomatic aspects of sexual dysfunction in males, not only in the case of PE, have often been observed. Quite often, such aspects remain non-reported, or remain unconscious. Thus, they have to be inferred from biographies of patients. More frequently in psychotherapeutic practice, the dysfunction itself is not reported at first but only later in the therapeutic process. It is not rare to see an interactional etiology even before the symptom has been described. Sexual dysfunction very often has an interactional etiology and always interactional consequences. Although sometimes denied or trivialized, after all, potency is always a male issue. Anamnestic questionnaires can tell about that. Dysfunction does emerge, whether patients are circumcised or not. Yet, myths and beliefs of circumcision as a measure that might reduce potency gives an idea that there are fantasies of all kinds toward circumcision. Moreover, circumcision is not widespread in northern European countries (which are here referred to as European countries northern of the Alpes), and this survey is to reintroduce reasonable dealings with the topic.

Physiology and pathophysiology in penile erection can be viewed in many publications; detailed overviews of its mechanisms have been given [8], and contexts of psychosomatic interconnections have broadened the perspective (cf. [10]). Many publications have given elaborate overviews of clinical management of male sexual function (cf. [11]). Especially in PE, there are many research results and management approaches of which excellent surveys have been published (cf. [12]). As can be seen, the prevalence of PE in the world's middle-east region is less than half (12.4%) of the average (somewhere between 27.4 and 30.5%) in other regions of the world [12]. The question must be raised whether this is merely an artifact or not. Why, will be discussed further below. In the following chapters, a closer look at circumcision from different perspectives is to broaden the view of sexual dysfunction and PE. After public opinion aspects at first, psychological and clinical aspects of circumcision and associated subjects follow some practice study data. As in most research from non-exact sciences, such as the disciplines related to humanities, it has to be clear that anything dealing with psyche will sometimes be hypothetical, or even speculative. Aspects discussed below cannot be depicted in their entirety but only as consistent as possible. There may be arguments against some of them. Further research would be welcome at any rate.

2. Public opinion

Circumcision as a minor medical practice in northern Europe had not been a highly crucial topic in public opinion until 2012, when a German minor regional court verdict on circumcision without medical indication was published [13]. The verdict that would have prohibited circumcision solely on behalf of cultural, religious, hygienic, or aesthetic reasons and in favor of medical reasons only led to a broad debate in the public as well as to its overturn and to a regulation of law by the end of 2012, all the more legalizing circumcision, albeit with some minor requirements (overview in Ref. [14]). German-speaking media had only occasionally reported on this issue, yet discussions emerged on the Internet (in Austria, e.g., on net-doktor.at). In times of increasing genital surgery in women, for example, labioplastics [15], the so-called designer's vagina [16], and along the trend of increasing intimacy in public perception it might be true that also the northern European population took on body modification options that might have led to wishing to have the penile foreskin removed more often than before. Increasing parts of the European population, for whatever reasons cannot be discussed here, have come to favor total depilization of pubic hair, having intimate tattoos and piercings. On the one hand, in northern countries there has been a general rejection especially as to newborn and infant circumcision; on the other hand an ongoing trend in modifying one's body parts seems to have triggered more people's interest in influences from southern cultural regions, particularly the Jewish, Muslim, or American sphere. The impression that circumcision even in German everyday life is more frequent than assumed initiated taking a further look at the subject.

3. Practice study data

A spontaneous screening of patients' mothers (aged 23–43) in a German urban practice for integrative gynecological psychosomatics and psychotherapy of children and adolescents, asking for early child illness and medical intervention data, revealed that 60% (12; $n = 20$) of their sons (aged 5–14) had been circumcised. This seems to be a very high percentage that no one would have expected. Only 25% (5) of the patients were of Muslim migration families, 10% (2) were of German-American background. Out of five German patients' mothers who had their sons circumcised, two declared phimosis as the reason, and three ticked other reasons (e.g., aesthetic and hygienic) (cf. [14]). This being a small, non-representative sample may not carry statistical evidence, yet in the context of societal trends it hints at the current development of migration and on collective fantasies about aesthetics, hygiene, and sexuality. Before the start of the practice study, there had been an informal exchange with a German child surgeon and an Austrian urologist, the latter stating circumcision in Austria to have a much better reputation than in Germany, emphasizing that the rate of circumcisions in Austria definitely was increasing. Some counter-movements are certainly existent too, igniting the debate on circumcision every now and then. This has been the case in the US and in Germany in a debate on bodily integrity, in Germany rather with an emphasis on nature orientation. Some medical circles refer to self-imposed imperatives of nature orientation as "German frenzy of naturalness" [17]. However, a way too anxious labeling of circumcision as psychic trauma ought to be withstood; all too excessively the term trauma has been psychologically applied on any given medical event. Empathic presence of parents prevents children from traumatic experiencing of painful events (cf. [18, 19]), and the cultural anticipation of an intervention is most crucial [20]. Not circumcision itself, but its handling in the family, their communication, and their emotions about it seem to be pivotal to dealing with it. Case studies have occasionally pointed that out (e.g., [21]).

4. Psychological aspects

From a historical mentality point of view, it is fair to state that in the majority of Europe's Christian occidental heritage countries, along the nineteenth and early twentieth century nature movement and the so-called youth movement [Jugendbewegung], as well as especially in Germany's experience of the Nazi Regime and the execution of genocide, there has come to exist a strong collective affect against violations of bodily integrity. In the course, recent popular reports on female genital mutilation practices have oddly transformed into some general equation with male circumcision, some of them revealing horrendous ignorance of anatomy. By that, any Jewish or Muslim family involuntarily came to be on the brink of general suspicion of executing violent educational modes. This has to be critically reflected since any reflex of demonizing circumcision is not only beyond reason; possibly it rather serves as a psychic displacement of general socio-political issues toward a minor medical issue. Reports of children's poverty in Germany show outrageous rates although the children's rights movement has long reached policy-makers. In a country with very high average incomes and high gross national product, this seems like oddly displacing societal issues toward a minor surgical operation.

Here, we elaborate on why mostly in northern European countries in public opinion circumcision still is often rejected or has an at least questionable reputation and why advocators of circumcision tend to be viewed as non-empathic, if not sadistic aggressors. Pondering these issues does not refer to the pros and cons of ritual infant circumcision; what is at stake here is the psychic fantasy about removing the prepuce in general. As said before, this tradition has especially been practiced regularly in Jewish, Muslim, and Anglo-American cultures. Interestingly enough, Judaism and Islam are the two world religions that are related to Christianity the most (cf. [22]). Cultural differences between the latter have first of all emerged from secularization, which has different concepts and facets. Whereas, for example, in secular Islamic countries, there has been a segregation of religion from worldly life and from the state—which is the laicist version—in Christianity secularization rather means having worldly life permeated by religion. Christian secularization is thus different from Jewish or Islamic secularization: it means religion is confounded with worldly life, and not worldly life averting religion [23]. The differences in countries conducting secularization have been large; for example, France, or the US, being strictly laicist whereas, for example, Germany is not.

The whole history of circumcision cannot be depicted here; recently, a concise and informing overview has been published [24]. The pivotal issue is whether specifically the Christian ambivalence of sexuality is responsible for even secularized northern European citizens so to reject and dismiss circumcision in general. Much of the uttered care in the debate on bodily integrity actually does not seem to play much of a role in, for example, tonsillectomy. This is why it can be useful to explore passed-by images and fantasies from the cultural sphere where they stem from. What might a circumcised male represent in the fantasies of people from these countries? He might have been fantasied as a sexually potent man. On a visual level, showing the glans penis in contrast to covering it may give a sexually aggressive, which means potent, impression. In flaccid state, the glans would be concealed in uncircumcised men until in erected state, so that the visual difference is physically entrenched in the circumcised organ. So it is the visual impression which is a factor and which finds its deposit psychic. Taking into consideration Norbert Elias' theory of a steadily increasing civilizational process in history [25], it is fair to say that in ancient times highly aggressive interactional behavior would be as common in everyday issues as in sexual issues. Psychic defense and coping mechanisms like, for example, sublimation would develop only late in human history as cultural-processing modes that were at the same time founding and requiring more complex societies. Taking into account the concept of educational modes [26] with ubiquitous infanticidal modes reaching back to ancient times, it becomes clear that—apart from the ever-existing exceptions of small elite groups—in common dealings there would be quite a coarse and brutal daily routine. Sexual matters would not be excluded from that way of living. Neither phenomena of industrial society like the decrease in sperm count nor lack of testosterone in men are likely to have existed—again, with the exception of the ever-present single cases. The common perception of males will have been a perception of being coarse and brute, not like in supposable idealized artistic or religious depictions. Along the civilizational development, and along enlightenment and humanistic influences on everyday dealings, people became more structured, became tamer, and became more orderly, this of course taking its toll in loss of spontaneity and directness. The mental process of sublimation, for example, directing of libidinous energy toward socially acceptable goals [27], probably became more prominent in the western world only from the eighteenth century on (violent regressions in war as contra-directional tendency being its inherent, dialectic counterpart). So in different periods, different modes of personalities and their dealings with one another would exist, developing in a long process toward—relatively—more peaceful and equanimous personalities. With that, along the twentieth century even gender roles became blurred, so that only at the turn of the millennium to the twenty-first century, going along with post-feminism, females could enjoy the freedom struggled for endlessly. Last but not least, through reintroducing of further accentuation of female sexual stimuli (e.g., aesthetic surgery), males got to be perceived as more male, and masculinity is more required than before. Even movies and television tell about that trend (cf. [28]), so that the sexes, in terms of male-female differentiation, are tending to be relocated at classic concept (gender issues otherwise becoming even more important, what is not necessarily in contradiction to increasing male-female differentiation). Viewed from a psychobiological perspective, this is to be welcomed. Significantly, the current trend toward re-appreciating of male aspects in men goes along with the accentuation of female aspects in women. This can serve as a psychobiological rationale of the visual, psychic perception of males, and it might entail a new trend toward circumcision. Moreover, oriental habits and customs have encompassed each and every erogenous zone of the human body, while through the influence of Christian churches especially in western Europe such dealings have remained unusual [29]—even when there have been many changes. However, in ancient times, a circumcised penis would necessarily draw attention and trigger rejection or fascination, at any rate trigger reaction at all. It seems clear that the glans penis visible hints at the erectibility of the penis [24], fitting it out with more of a specific sexual note in contrast to an uncircumcised penis. The fact that in Christian-heritage art the penis is depicted smaller than it is in reality [30] is an indication of Christian disesteem, too. The point is, in psychic reality, what is called "the other" is often tainted with defect, that is, what has been unknown will trigger discontent; certainly a fact in the perception of difference in the circumcision debate (cf. [31]).

Perhaps more important than appearance, the issue of the presence of a so-called paternal principle might relate to it, that is, circumcision as a symbolic act of castration by the father. Seemingly odd, circumcision as a symbolic castration would differentiate the man from the boy. To be a man, one would have to go through circumcision first. By contrast, an uncircumcised man would be no more than a big boy who did not undergo incest taboo and some other rules and regulations that come along with the concept of Nom-du-Père, that is, the law-, or name-of-the-father (Lacan, cf. [32]). This concept of Nom-du-Père manifests itself in the actual cutting of the penile foreskin, this being an act of transforming the penis into a phallus. Apart from the ancient notion of the phallus symbolizing power, fertility, and death-defiance, the idea is to declare and maintain paternal parentage, which cannot be testified through human senses (cf. [33]). However, witness can historically testify maternal descent. Thus, maternal parentage is obvious and visible, and in the course of their development it has to be psychically dismissed by males. Accepting and overcoming it at the same time is pivotal to male identity development. So, roughly speaking, in order to become a man in their own right, males have to partially relinquish female lines of identification. What Freud on a macro-level described as renunciation of sensuality in favor of an advance in intellectuality in Judaism [34] on a micro-level finds its analogy in male development. This process is attested by circumcision, which leaves a visible trace of this process. It also testifies incompleteness and vulnerability of the male body, which in females is naturally symbolized by menstruation [23]. As can be seen, here we have a connection between Islam and Judaism, which is also true for the differentiation of the sexes and their symbolic order. As to such an order, in practice looking at today's northern European patient families, it is not far-fetched to state that quite frequently hardly any paternal principle has been established. Surprisingly enough, in terms of the sample data above, several young German-based mothers now seem to symbolically establish a paternal principle substitute by having their sons circumcised. This might be understood as a symbolic act of anticipating, or making up ritual, of their individuation toward manhood.

Last but not least, the myth of circumcision for deterring masturbation (which of course can be traced to a large amount of sources) might be a myth itself. Unconsciously, advocators of circumcision in history might have considered masturbation itself not so much of a problem, but might have considered masturbation with prepuce a problem. Why? Because it literally can be regarded as having sexual intercourse with oneself. It tends to an even more inert and uncreative handling of sexuality. Back in time, circumcision advocators might intuitively have figured out right that disturbances of the senses will be triggered even more through stimulating the penis with an artificial meatus, which the prepuce would be, tending to replace objectal stimulation through the anatomy of a sexual partner by subjectal stimulation through one's own anatomy. So what may sound far-fetched at first might have an unconscious foundation in grasping a real-life issue. This is not to say that masturbation is generally bad: as always in medical issues, dose makes the poison; it is but a secondary means of handling sexuality.

5. Clinical aspects

Although hardly any disadvantages of circumcision have been reported [35, 36], every now and then, in medical publications invectives against it emerge, sometimes from a pediatric, sometimes from an alternative, rarely from a gynecological background. At the same time, in scientific urological and sexual medical journals more often than not, functional, hygienic, and sexual advantages after circumcision are reported. Apparently, increasing parts of medical circles consider circumcisions making sense on different levels. Facts and necessities of circumcision are regularly depicted there, as, for example, in balanitis, in lichen sclerosus, in preventing of infections of different kinds [37–39], of penile carcinoma [40, 41], or in a possible decrease of cervical carcinoma in females [36, 42, 43], this even in traditionally noninvasive German complementary and alternative medical publications [44, 45]. Claude Bernard's motto, germs are nothing, substrate is everything, seems to be reintroduced by now (quoted in [46]). Prognostically, a further increase of circumcisions in northern Europe is highly probable, not only for migration reasons but also for globalizing of aesthetic practices reasons. Whereas British pediatricians now tend to dismiss routine infant circumcision, American physicians keep on advocating it quite generally [47–49]. Nowadays, most clinicians would not remove an appendix or the tonsils prophylactically. A conservative, noninvasive stance may definitely be right, and experienced clinicians know very well when to intervene and when not. At any rate, it does not seem to be appropriate to make the prepuce a fetish and transform it into a signifier of health and happiness, as has often been done in northern Europe. Especially, anxiety of suture and of keloid scars seems to be in the way, although these are issues which have come to be handled well [50]. Of course, climate conditions play a role: the climate in northern Europe is not the same as it is in, for example, the Alpe-Adria region, let alone in the Mediterranean and further into more southern regions. Of course, hot and humid climates support generating of some bacteria and microorganisms. By 1962, research findings compared the small amount of germs in a circumcised penis to that of an uncircumcised penis with a condom on [51], something that would be conclusive to generations of Americans. Some facts are not well known in northern Europe as yet: inflammation of the glans penis is not a rare event particularly in uncircumcised boys. Significantly, urinary tract infections in boys tend to be more frequent—up to 10 times—in the uncircumcised [52]; the risk of cervical carcinoma as to hygienic standard in Israel is 3.8 per 100,000, in Germany 16 per 100,000 [45]. The team of Castellsague et al. has elaborated on this, and Rivet in her stock-check has given a distinct account from a family physician's point of view [42, 43].

In the case of a female patient wishing for her partner's foreskin to be removed for hygienic reasons (cf. [14]), in a 2-year follow-up the couple confirmed refraining from relatively short cohabitation time periods of around 5–10 min they had before circumcision—except for when intended. Following that, the result was that after 2 years the patient's now-circumcised partner had gained more control of his sexual functioning. It must be added that in anamnesis, none of these issues had been issues at all, essentially since the patient had sought psychotherapy for different reasons. In retrospect, the couple had sexually been quite happy before, although the patient reported to have problems reaching orgasm every now and then. Following their statements, there had been a significant increase in satisfaction after circumcision. Subclinical as it may be the case points to an interesting hypothesis: female sexual dysfunction not only can have many facets in phenotype and in psychosomatic etiology aspects (cf. [6]) but, as to PE, female orgasm disorders well known in daily practice might at times be considered an artifact due to male PE. Complaints on cohabitation time periods of 1–2 min may be a disguised PE; here, possibly, a symptom of males is displaced toward females who present with orgasm disorders as an allegedly female issue [53]. At any rate, cohabitation time period in circumcised males is frequently assumed to be longer than in uncircumcised males. Although there has not been any consistent evidence so far, the Italian study might support the public opinion. Moreover, in a recent review on PE, the authors [54] put frenulum breve at anecdote category, oddly ignoring the Italian study. They attempt a hint at cultural differences in what qualifies as a symptom and what does not—what may generally be right but not applicable in all ways. In their review, PE is attributed to some patriarchal cultures, at the same time generally imputing low self-esteem to women from these cultures who will not tend to rate rapid ejaculation as premature but as a sign of male virility; that is why PE is not diagnosed. Rather, in some cases PE may not exist because of differing cultural scripts. What the authors seem to withhold is differing cultural scripts of sexual encounter which can be completely different. Such scripts can grossly differ from the majority of, say, western scripts. Scripts as subsequent oral or manual stimulation toward female orgasm, usually followed by a second, more lasting cohabitation act, have to be taken into consideration in order to approach reality proper. These are not even considered existent by the authors, let alone further examined. In orientalism, specific female vaginal or anal muscular techniques have been used to provoke rapid ejaculation in males. Multiple sexual acts are not only in opposition to PE functionally [55] but maybe even by definition, thus highly culturally dependent. Again, orientalism has produced different relations to bodily issues, such as sexuality [29]. This might confirm the data of low prevalence in the middle-east cited above [12] in a more appropriate way than coercing data into fitting culturally insensitive reasoning. Lately, a psychoanalytic account has been given of historical idealization, or special appreciation of sexuality in Islam in opposition to its perception in Christianity [56], which should be similar in Judaism. Of course, differentiations must be further examined (cf. [57]). All in all, psychogenic erectile dysfunction in general not only often has short duration [4] but especially in the case of PE is subjected to different cultural scripts that will influence, if not define, symptom formation.

Another case shows a male patient who presented with situative erectile dysfunction, with a more complex psychosomatic background. The patient had a history of fantasying about his urethra carrying residue of urine mingling with his sperm when ejaculating, something that in his opinion would be a hygienic problem. His idea was that fluids must not mingle. He reported that this idea had bothered him ever since he was sexually active. He had been circumcised at the age of 4, and he could not remember to have had any problems about it. In sexual situations with his partner and with ex-partners in the past, he felt disgusted that they did not share his view but even enjoyed active oral sex. He had been with his current partner for 2 years, and she had assured him not to have any problem with his theory of fluids, and as a biology student she was right, he admitted. During coitus, he usually felt like having to ejaculate prematurely which in reality he did not. However, he would mentally keep on being sexually excited while his erection would be waning. Only through further active stimulation by his partner would he be able to continue, which for him felt like starting anew. Such an interactional loop could take place several times a night. The therapeutic process led to joint understanding of the patient's fantasies behind the symptom, of his feeling of nausea over smegma, of his theory of fluids that revealed a strict dichotomy between good and bad, and the like. Moreover, it led to the conclusion that his psychogenic dysfunction was somewhat linked to circumcision. It was the patient himself who suggested to view his sexual mode of behavior as some kind of pseudo-premature ejaculation, and he referred to an uncircumcised friend of his who was under treatment with PE diagnosis. After having reported to him about his ideas of hygiene, the friend told him about having a smegma problem although applying steady hygienic measures. The patient remembered to have heard of such a problem a long time ago. In the process of time, it had added to no more than severe qualms about his self-confidence, which took 3 years to be reestablished. What was surprisingly easy to handle was the erectile dysfunction he had since in his mind, he felt like uncircumcised. Still in the end, it was not so much bibliotherapy that accounted for an alleviation of his dysfunction but, apart from the ever-effective therapeutic alliance, it was his realizing of the fact that he had been circumcised which made him comfortable with himself. The points his partner had made, such as dryness of the glans, would make him easy with his genital in contrast to the friend of his who at his wife's behest would have to clean his penis twice a day. Through less than a few months period, his concept of hygiene was waning while his erection would come back, and his fantasy to ejaculate early lost its urge. If the patient had not been circumcised the case would have been different and have led to even more complex entanglement—given the patient would have had the same fantasies anyway. In a 1-year-catamnestic questionnaire, the patient reported of no more dysfunction during the act, and his partner and himself described cohabitation quality and quantity as excellent. What is even more significant is, there would not be any displacement of symptom toward dysmorphophobia, something that by all means might have been the case. In this case, as to psychosomatic symptom formation, the sexual dysfunction had been a highly limited and well-accessible symptom.

Even when some research is limited, one can examine sexual functioning and experiencing of patients. As to functioning, the point is that erection is controlled by mechanisms in the hypothalamus, cerebral cortex, and spinal cord. Most important is the neural control of erection, which is organized afferently and efferently. In afferent direction, infraspinal and supraspinal influences on the spinal erection center can trigger erection. In reflexogenic erection, afferences extend via the pudendal nerve toward the sacral erection center which sends out efferences via the plexus hypogastricus inferior. In psychogenic erection, sensory, visual, or acoustic stimuli or fantasies trigger erection, with the involvement of cortical centers. In efferent direction, stimulation of the autonomous nervous system triggers erection, influencing penile vessels. The parasympathetic nervous system is pro-erectile; the sympathetic is anti-erectile. Penile vessels are innervated by preganglionic neurons in the spinal cord. Innervation runs via the plexus hypogastricus inferior and cavernosi nerves toward the penile corpus cavernosum. From the sacral plexus on, the pudendal nerve innervates pelvic musculature; pelvic floor contraction intensifies rigidity. After all, erection can be described as a neurovascular event involving sensory, motor, and autonomous nerves. Cavernosal structures and blood circulation in the penis are involved, as are hormones and neurotransmitters. Apart from molecular signal transduction which has been depicted extensively [8], sexual experiencing plays another important role. It will find its deposit psychically, as psyche will have predetermined experiencing and with that nerve system parameters.

Penile nerve supply is essentially conducted by the compact twin dorsal penile nerves which emerge from under the pubic bone. Running toward the glans, the nerve fibers fan out. Interestingly, although by circumcision corpuscular receptors of touch are removed, a recent sensory testing study found no long-term implications for penile sensitivity in circumcised males and even challenges the image of the foreskin to be the most sensitive part of the penis [48]. It is rather that, due to circumcision, loss of sensitivity of the glans as a result of keratinization will handicap ejaculation. Circumcision can stifle PE induced by high stimulation in the glans, or induced by high friction of the prepuce when in rhythmic contact with the glans in uncircumcised males.

Treatment of PE can be difficult, still behavioral and pharmacological approaches, and combinations of these, have often proven helpful. While PDE-5 inhibitors sustain penile erection and facilitate further sexual acts, they may support overcoming of anxiety that often exacerbates PE ([58], cf. [12]). Such additional effects are welcome in case of an indication of PDE-5 inhibitors. Some patients with psychosomatic involvement will benefit from a combination of pharmacotherapy and psychotherapy without too much of behavioral instruction. Psychodynamic examination of personal biography can produce good results. Still, behavioral approaches and cognitive therapy are useful, especially those that will reach both cognition and emotion in patients. Apart from well-known sexual behavioral therapy publications, it is interesting to see that behavioral therapy publications on depression and addiction have proven helpful ([59, 60] and generally, [61]), which points to psychodynamic similarities of these disorders to some type of sexual dysfunction, such as psychosomatic PE. Additionally, learning of relaxation techniques [62, 63] can have strong effects on sexual behavior and experiencing.

6. Discussion

Were it not for some good reasons, one might consider the foreskin superfluous from the beginning: the idea of hygiene has a point in its own right. Yet, it may have protected the glans penis from brush and plants in ancient times. An ideology of naturalness should not overrule today's hygienic or medical aspects, though. PE, which is by no means a rare issue in men of heterogeneous age and descent, is now being treated more and more by use of selective serotonin reuptake inhibitors [SSRIs] (cf. [12]), such as dapoxetine, which is used as on-demand treatment. This means intervening in neurotransmitter metabolism, which some European patient groups tend to refrain from completely. A possible loss of libido has been discussed, yet with no clear conclusion. All in all, dapoxetine research results are remarkable and are open to debate. However, PE patients ought to be diagnosed thoroughly, and uncircumcised men ought to be counseled. It stands to reason that checking of physiological and psychological status should be first of all. Meticulously detailed anamnesis also of psychosocial biography is required, even via questionnaires quite analogous to those of different focus [64]. Instead of rapidly going for medication in times of high pressure, which seems to be the easiest option to some efficiency-oriented patients, an exact analysis of PE and related disorders will be most helpful. In PE, the frenulum breve study ought to trigger attention to circumcision as a possible first-line option, especially in case that a restrictive frenular band was not the rare anomaly but more usual than assumed while a sufficient one was the exception. It might as well be denied or trivialized, or be culturally experienced as normal. It may be that the frenulum interferes more with retraction of the prepuce than usually assumed. Especially as the prepuce is continuously retracted, which for reasons of hygiene has to be case, frequently reported minor tears can generate inelastic scar tissue and by further retracting of the prepuce generate even more tears and scars. Also, the size of the glans in relation to size and restrictiveness of the prepuce might generally be underrated as well. Further research is needed here.

Especially male patients do not tend to report voluntarily on pain, inflammation, or problems with the sexual act. They do almost only at request. Adolescent males will not easily admit to these problems, too. However, whereas in urological practices the elderly are by far the majority of patients, in Internet forums plenty of adolescents seem to appear with plenty of questions on genital function, dysfunction, and the like. While it has been confirmed that circumcision is not associated with higher prevalence of erectile dysfunction—as we have seen, the foreskin plays no important role in erectile function anyway [65]—PE has not been so much in public focus to date. In correspondence with the myth of circumcision to be a measure that affects potency or erection, it must be clear that there is still much information to be given to the northern European public. The fact that the Brookman May et al. study's authors declare their results to end a myth [3] is not for nothing: oddly telling, in the 2014 European Parliament election campaign, a German mock-party called Die Partei [66] even launched a poster which read, "Hände weg vom deutschen Pimmel!" ("Hands Off German Peter!"), ironically addressing western European bureaucratic standardization issues via the seemingly German anxiety of circumcision.

7. Conclusion

The sacredness of the female body in Judaism and Islam corresponds to circumcision in males, a cultural practice by which human incompleteness is written directly in the body. More important than tradition—which must always be questioned—is the aspect of symbolic order of the sexes that points to culturally dependent perception in general. Psychologically, anxiety might confirm circumcised males still to be fantasied as some sort of danger to the northern European Christian-heritage culture, even when this seems to be an ancient issue long ago. Still, ambivalence toward sexuality is a common topos in Christianity, whereas more openness toward sexuality in Judaism, in Islam, and in wide parts of Asia have been common. Due to its ethnic and cultural heterogeneity and its puritan heritage, the Anglo-American region seems to be somewhere in between.

As to the medical aspect of circumcision, no real adverse effects have been observed [36]. As to psychogenic PE, behavioral and pharmacological approaches should be augmented by detailed psychosomatic anamnesis. Circumcision may support alleviation in some cases. Generally, it seems that circumcision, in case it stands the test of time, will have to be dissociated from solely religious beliefs and unquestioned cultural traditions. Instead, a somewhat more reasonable approach would be useful in order to a get a grip on circumcision. Many gynecologists and urologists favor circumcision for good reasons.

Author details

Götz Egloff

Address all correspondence to: g.egloff.medpsych.ma@email.de

Practice for Psychoanalysis and Psychotherapy, Mannheim, affil, University of Heidelberg, Germany

References

[1] Gallo L, Perdonà S, Gallo A. The role of short frenulum and the effects of frenulectomy on premature ejaculation. Journal of Sexual Medicine. 2010;7(3):1269–1276

[2] Der Standard. Sep 6, 2011

[3] Brookman May S, Hoschke B, Fenske S, Pohling P, Spivak I, Gilfrich C, et al. Das Ende eines Mythos: Die männliche Zirkumzision ist nicht mit einer höheren Prävalenz der erektilen Dysfunktion assoziiert. Journal fur Urologie und Urogynakologie. 2014;**21**(2):12–16

[4] deMendonça RR, Korkes F, Zambon JP. Erectile dysfunction: Etiological factors. In: Nunes KP, editor. Erectile Dysfunction—Disease-Associated Mechanisms and Novel Insights into Therapy. Rijeka/Croatia: InTech Publisher; 2012. pp. 23–34

[5] Benedek T. Die Funktionen des Sexualapparates und ihre Störungen. In: Alexander F, editor. Psychosomatische Medizin. Berlin/New York: De Gruyter; 1985. pp. 170–210

[6] Egloff G. Wirklichkeiten und Möglichkeiten—analytisch-systemische Therapie einer 25-jährigen Klientin mit sexueller Funktionsstörung. Kontext. 2013;**44**(2):136–146

[7] Kuhl H. Sexualhormone und Psyche. Thieme: Stuttgart; 2002

[8] Nunes KP, Webb RC. Mechanisms in erectile function and dysfunction: An overview. In: Nunes KP, editor. Erectile Dysfunction—Disease-Associated Mechanisms and Novel Insights into Therapy. Rijeka/Croatia: InTech Publisher; 2012. pp. 3–22

[9] Egloff G. Potenz und Psyche: PDE-5-Hemmer als Low-dose-Dauermedikation? AZN Arzt, Zahnarzt und Naturheilverfahren. 2012;**12**(1):12–13

[10] Harth W. Psychosomatische Aspekte sexueller Funktionsstörungen. In: Harth W, Brähler E, Schuppe HC, editors. Praxishandbuch Männergesundheit. Berlin: Medizinisch Wissenschaftliche Verlagsgesellschaft; 2012. pp. 258–270

[11] Mulcahy JJ, editor. Male Sexual Function. A Guide to Clinical Management. New York: Springer; 2001

[12] Al-Shaiji TF. Premature ejaculation revisited: Definition and contemporary management approaches. In: Nunes KP editor. Erectile Dysfunction—Disease-Associated Mechanisms and Novel Insights into Therapy. Rijeka/Croatia: InTech Publisher; 2012. pp. 97–126

[13] Ärzte-Zeitung. June 28, 2012

[14] Peschel P, Egloff G. Zirkumzision in Deutschland—männliche Beschneidung mit Rechtssicherheit? gyne. 2012;**33**(12):22–24

[15] Brandenburg U. Lifting für die Schamlippen. gynäkologie + geburtshilfe. 2009;**14**(12): 32

[16] Hohl MK., Scheidel P, Schüssler B. Designer-Vagina. Frauenheilkunde Aktuell. 2008;**17**(1): 4–14

[17] Wiegratz I, Kuhl H. Langzyklus. Thieme: Stuttgart; 2010.

[18] Bachhofen A. Heile Welten. Der unbewusste Verzicht der Kriegsenkel auf ein eigenes Leben. In: Knoch H, Kurth W., Reiss HJ, Egloff G, editors. Die Kinder der Kriegskinder und die späten Folgen des NS-Terrors. Heidelberg: Mattes; 2012. pp. 101–112

[19] Bachhofen A. Trauma und Beziehung. Grundlagen eines intersubjektiven Behandlungsansatzes. Stuttgart: Klett-Cotta; 2012

[20] Morris BJ, Waskett JH, Banerjee J, Wamai RG, Tobian AAR, Gray RH, et al. A 'snip' in time: What is the best age to circumcise? BMC Pediatrics. 2012;**12**:20

[21] Egloff G, Becker B. Defizit- und Lösungsorientierung in der systemischen Psychotherapie. Chancen und Gefahren am Beispiel der Einzeltherapie eines 32-jährigen Patienten mit depressiven und aggressiven Tendenzen. CoMed. 2011;**18**(3):66–69

[22] Bertau K. Schrift—Macht—Heiligkeit in den Literaturen des jüdisch-christlich-muslimischen Mittelalters. Hg. Sonja Glauch. Berlin/New York: De Gruyter; 2005

[23] von Braun C. Die symbolische Geschlechterordnung in den drei Religionen des Buches—Säkularisierung und Post-Sexualität. Sexuologie. 2016;**23**(1-2):39–47

[24] Hafner G. Zirkumzision—der Schnitt in den Knaben. Sexuologie. 2012;**19**(1-2):9–17

[25] Elias N. Über den Prozess der Zivilisation. Soziogenetische und psychogenetische Untersuchungen. Vols. 1 & 2. Frankfurt: Suhrkamp; 1997

[26] deMause L. The Emotional Life of Nations. New York: Karnac; 2002

[27] Freud S. Drei Abhandlungen zur Sexualtheorie. GW, Vol. 5. Frankfurt: Fischer; 1905/1999

[28] Egloff G, Gioeni P. Einbruch des Eros—Black Swan als psychosexueller Entwicklungsroman. In: Langendorf U, Kurth W, Reiss HJ, Egloff G. editors. Gespaltene Gesellschaft und die Zukunft von Kindheit. Heidelberg: Mattes; 2013. pp. 263–282

[29] Rieger B. Die Prostata. Munich: Herbig; 2009

[30] Lippert H. Lehrbuch Anatomie. 5th ed. Munich: Urban & Fischer; 2000. pp. 426–430

[31] Çetin Z, Wolter SA. Fortsetzung einer "Zivilisierungsmission": Zur deutschen Beschneidungsdebatte. In: Çetin Z, Voss HJ, Wolter SA , editors. Interventionen gegen die deutsche Beschneidungsdebatte. Münster: Edition Assemblage; 2012. pp. 15–50

[32] Fink B. Einführung in die Lacansche Psychoanalyse. Vienna: Turia & Kant; 2009

[33] Rickels LA. Die Unterwelt der Psychoanalyse. Vienna: Passagen; 2014. pp. 35–41

[34] Freud S. Der Mann Moses und die monotheistische Religion. StA, Vol. 9. Frankfurt: Fischer; 1939/1974. p. 557

[35] Schoen EJ. Male circumcision. In: Kandeel FR, Lue TF, Pryor JL, Swerdloff RS editors. Male Sexual Dysfunction. Pathophysiology and Treatment. Informa, New York; 2007. pp. 95–107

[36] Morris BJ, Wodak AD, Mindel A, Schrieber L, Duggan KA, Dilley A, et al. Infant male circumcision: An evidence-based policy statement. Open Journal of Preventive Medicine. 2012;**2**(1):2–24

[37] Tobian AAR, Serwadda D, Quinn TC, Kigozi G, Gravitt PE, Laeyendecker O, et al. Male circumcision for the prevention of HSV-2, HPV and syphilis. The New England Journal of Medicine. 2009;**360**:1298–1309

[38] Scola N, Altmeyer P, Kreuter A. Lichen sklerosus, Diagnostik und Therapie einer oft übersehenen Erkrankung. gyne. 2012;**33**(6):20–22

[39] Schwarz T. Extravaginale Reservoire für die bakterielle Vaginose verantwortlich. gynäkologie + geburtshilfe. 2012;**17**(6):16

[40] Köhn FM, Pflieger Bruss S, Schill WB. Penile skin diseases. Andrologia. 1999;**31**:3–11

[41] Köhn FM. Dermatosen des männlichen Genitales. In: Harth W, Brähler E, Schuppe HC. editors. Praxishandbuch Männergesundheit. Berlin: Medizinisch Wissenschaftliche Verlagsgesellschaft; 2012. pp. 206–213

[42] Castellsague X, Bosch X, Munoz N, Meijer CJLM, Shah KV, De Sanjose S, et al. Male circumcision, penile human papillomavirus infection, and cervical cancer in female partners. New England Journal of Medicine. 2002;**346**:1105–1112

[43] Rivet C. Circumcision and cervical cancer. Is there a link? Canadian Family Physician. 2003;**49**:1096–1097

[44] Herzog A. Die Impfung gegen das Zervixkarzinom. Forum Komplementäre Onkologie. 2011;**1**:9–11

[45] Herzog A. Präventionsmassnahme beim Cervixkarzinom—Impfung sinnvoll oder Geldverschwendung? Praxis Magazin. 2011;**28**(5):16–19

[46] Schwarz P. Vaginalmykosen—Innovativer Ansatz zur Prävention und Therapie. CoMed. 2012;**19**(4):63–67

[47] Canadian Pediatric Society. Neonatal circumcision revisited. Fetus and Newborn Committee. Canadian Medical Association Journal. 1996;**154**(6):769–780

[48] Bossio JA, Pukall CF, Steele SS. Examining penile sensitivity in neonatally circumcised and intact men using quantitative sensory testing. Journal of Urology. 2016;**195**(6):1848–1853

[49] American College of Obstetricians and Gynecologists. Male circumcision. Pediatrics. 2012;**130**(3):756–786

[50] Beller KD, Friedrich M. Schneller zu schöneren Narben—Möglichkeiten der Narbenbehandlung. Praxis Magazin. 2004;**21**(4):14–17

[51] Stern P, Neely PM. Cancer of the cervix in reference to circumcision and marital history. Journal of the American Medical Women's Association. 1962;**17**(9):738–740

[52] Voss HJ. Zirkumzision—die deutsche Debatte und ihre medizinische Basis. Sexuologie. 2012;**19**(3-4):154–162

[53] Bragagna E. Der weibliche Orgasmus—jenseits von Mythen. gynäkologie + geburtshilfe. 2013;**18**(5):28–31

[54] Buntrock S, Rösing D. Die Ejaculatio Praecox in sexualmedizinischer Theorie und Praxis. Sexuologie. 2014;**21**(1-2):63–75

[55] McMahon CG. Etiology and management of premature ejaculation. Nature Clinical Practice Urology. 2005;**2**(9):426–433

[56] Jiko J. Die Idealisierung des sexuellen Triebes im Islam. Psyche—Z Psychoanal. 2007;**61**:1132–1154

[57] Schneider I. Der Islam und die Frauen. Munich: C.H. Beck; 2011

[58] Sadeghi Nejad H, Watson R. Premature ejaculation: Current medical treatment and new directions. Journal of Sexual Medicine. 2008;**5**(5):1037–1050

[59] Beck AT, Rush AJ., Shaw BF, Emery G. Kognitive Therapie der Depression. Weinheim: Beltz/PVU; 1996

[60] Beck AT, Wright FD, Newman CF, Liese BS. Kognitive Therapie der Sucht. Weinheim: Beltz/PVU; 1997

[61] Walen SR., diGiuseppe R, Wessler RL. RET-Training. Munich: Pfeiffer; 1982.

[62] Bernstein DA, Borkovec TD. Entspannungstraining—Handbuch der progressiven Muskelentspannung. Munich: Pfeiffer; 1997

[63] Pierre Simon Laplace University, editor. Progressive Muskelentspannung nach Jacobson. Lenz/Switzerland: Trainermanual; 1997

[64] Barrett B, Lewis RW, Terris MK, Moses KA. Designing the rehabilitation of men with post-prostatectomy erectile dysfunction using a pre- and post-operative approach. Journal of Andrology & Gynaecology. 2013;**1**(1):6

[65] Lue TF. Physiology of penile erection and pathophysiology of erectile dysfunction and priapism. In: Walsh PC, Retik AB, Vaughan FD, Wein AJ, editors. Campbell's Urology. Saunders, Philadelphia; 1998. pp. 1157–1180

[66] Die Partei. Hände weg vom deutschen Pimmel! Poster, European Parliament Election Campaign; 2014